VIRAL HEPATITIS - SELECTED ISSUES OF PATHOGENESIS AND DIAGNOSTICS

Edited by **Sergey L. Mukomolov**

Viral Hepatitis - Selected Issues of Pathogenesis and Diagnostics
Edited by Sergey L. Mukomolov

Published by InTech

Janeza Trdine 9, 51000 Rijeka, Croatia

Publishing Process Manager Adriana Pecar

Technical Editor Teodora Smiljanic

Cover Designer InTech Design Team

Additional hard copies can be obtained from orders@intechopen.com

Viral Hepatitis - Selected Issues of Pathogenesis and Diagnostics,
Edited by Sergey L. Mukomolov
p. cm.
ISBN 978-953-307-760-4

For EU product safety concerns:
IN TECH d.o.o., Prolaz Marije Krucifikse Kozulić 3, 51000 Rijeka, Croatia,
info@intechopen.com or visit our website at intechopen.com.

Meet the editor

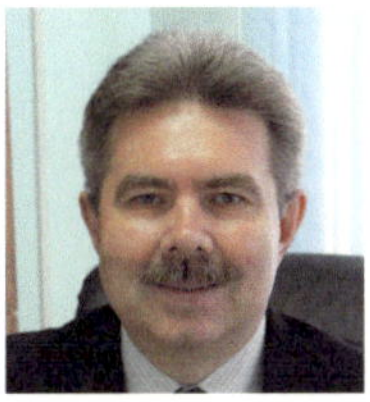

Professor Sergey L. Mukomolov MD, PhD, DSc is the Head of Epidemiology department and Viral hepatitis Laboratory in Saint-Petersburg Pasteur Institute. He is also a professor in Tropical Medicine department at North-Western State medical university named after I.I.Mechnikov. He started his professional career in 1981 after graduating from Leningrad (now Saint-Petersburg, Russia) medical university. His first PhD thesis (1984) was focused on clinical and epidemiological features of chronic Hepatitis B virus carriers; second one (1994) discussed the acute and chronic Hepatitis C viral infection. Now professor Mukomolov is one of the leading researchers in the field of diagnostics, epidemiology and prevention of viral hepatitis in the Russian Federation. He is the author of 230 publications and inventor of 7 patents. The results of his most important studies were published in well known journals like Journal of Viral Hepatitis, Journal of Virology, Journal of Medical Virology and many others.

Contents

Preface

There are five main causative agents of viral hepatitis, referred to as hepatitis viruses type A, B, C, D and E (HAV, HBV, HCV, HDV, HEV). These five viruses are of greatest concern because of the burden of illness and death.

In according to World Health Organization (WHO) about 2 billion people worldwide have been infected with the HBV and about 350 million live with chronic infection. It is estimated that 600 000 persons die each year due to the acute or chronic consequences of hepatitis B: liver cirrhosis and cancer. Furthermore, it is estimated that 3–4 million people are infected with the HCV each year. 130–170 million people are chronically infected with HCV and at risk of developing liver cirrhosis and/or liver cancer. More than 350 000 people die from HCV-related liver diseases each year. Statistically, 60–70% of HCV chronically-infected persons develop chronic liver disease, 5-20% develop cirrhosis and 1–5% die from cirrhosis or liver cancer.

Another big problem is related to fecal-orally transmitted HAV and HEV. The course of these two diseases is always acute and it does not lead to form chronic complications. However, we should remember; it is estimated that annually 1.4 milion cases of HAV infections is detected worldwide. Epidemics related to contaminated food or water can erupt explosively, such as an epidemic in Shanghai in 1988 that affected about 300 000 people. A mix HAV infection with chronic HBV or HCV related diseases could be lethal for patient.

During the last years researchers have paid more attention to the HEV infection due to its appearance in non-endemic areas (like Europe for example) and a probable link to development of chronic liver disease.

There are a lot of important issues regarding the viral hepatitis which needed to be studied: molecular biology of viruses, laboratory diagnostics, epidemiology, treatment etc. Special textbooks and monographs about these issues were published over the last decades. Taking in account this fact and rather fast progress in our understanding of the problem, the aim of our book is to focus on the important sections of the problem – immune pathogenesis of parenterally transmitted viral hepatitis and some aspects of hepatitis diagnostics.

Seven chapters were prepared (by several groups of researchers) to share information and results of studies with specialists who work in the field of viral hepatitis and persons who are interested to learn about this problem.

Dr Juan R Larrubia and his co-authors discuss the innate and adaptive immunity in the first chapter of the book entitled "HBV & HCV Immunopathogenesis". The separate section of this chapter covers humoral and cellular response in case of acute and chronic HBV infection. It is emphasized that the specific CTLs play a central role in HBV&HCV immunopathogenesis. These cells are able to kill some infected hepatocytes inducing a minor liver damage, but also they secrete type-I cytokines responsible for non-cytopathic virus clearing.

The next chapter prepared by Prof. Joerg F. Schlaak et al. focuses on the role of local innate immunity of the liver in the pathogenesis of chronic viral hepatitis. Activation of the Toll-like receptors (TLR) system leads to the expression of pro-inflammatory (IL-6, IL-12, TNF-α) as well as anti-inflammatory cytokines (IL-10) by responsive cell types. TLR7, -8 and -9 additionally initiate Interferon-α (IFN-α) expression after binding of their specific ligands. The authors separately discuss HBV, HCV and HDV innate immunity as well as peculiarities of immune response in case of co-infection of HBV and HCV. It was suspected that therapeutic manipulations of the hepatic TLR pathways are of high interest for the development of novel treatment strategies.

These treatment strategies for viral hepatitis based on the immunopathogenesis knowledge are discussed in the chapter by Dr. Yukihiro Shimizu. The author discusses the developing of an optimal strategy to stimulate antiviral immune response with therapeutic potential, extensive analyses of immune mechanisms for successful viral eradication and immunosuppressive mechanisms induced by viral infection during persistent infection are required. These points are discussed at the beginning of the chapter, then followed by a discussion of immunotherapeutic approaches in both animal models and humans in the end.

Dr. Costin Streba and co-authors consider pathogenesis of chronic hepatitis as the complete interaction between stress, neuroimmunomodulation and ultimately the onset and progress of viral infections. The influence of the endocrine response systems, such as the hypothalamic-pituitary-adrenal axis (HPA) or the sympathetic-adrenal-medullary (SAM) on the end function and outcome of the immune response are discussed in the chapter.

Dr Josh Levitsky and Dr Lisa B. VanWagner rise a problem of viral hepatitis in the solid organ transplant recipients. The most important infectious agents which are frequent in allograft recipients are HBV and HCV. In addition, HEV is emerging as an increasing cause of chronic hepatitis and even cirrhosis whilst HDV plays an important role in both co-infection and superinfection of HBV in solid organ transplant recipients in industrialized countries. This chapter focuses primarily on the epidemiology, transmission, clinical presentation and management of the primary hepatitis viruses following solid organ transplantation.

The last two chapters cover fecal-orally transmitted HAV and HEV.

The chapter on hepatitis A infection prepared by Dr. Zahid Hussain is mostly concentrated on clinical course, epidemiology and molecular characteristics of the HAV. It is emphasized that the changes in epidemiological pattern would increase the disease burden. They may cause large community outbreaks and lead to increased healthcare cost.

Prof. Zhang Jingqiang and co-authors share the results of their studies on structure and function of the HEV capsid protein. These studies using cryo-EM and X-ray crystallography techniques, with a variety of biochemical studies, have provided a detailed picture of HEV-LP formed by the expressed capsid protein. These architectures shed light on the understanding of the function of capsid such as the assembly mechanism of icosohedarl capsid, virus infection and antibody interaction.

While preparing our book for print, we heard that the Nobel Prize Committee (field of physiology and medicine- year 2011) awarded Bruce A. Beutler and Jules A. Hoffmann *"for their discoveries concerning the activation of innate immunity"* whilst Ralph M. Steinman received an award *"for his discovery of the dendritic cell and its role in adaptive immunity"*. We are proud to say that our book is in line with these discoveries, because 3 chapters cover the problems of innate and adaptive immune response in case of viral hepatitis.

Professor Sergey L. Mukomolov
Head, Viral Hepatitis Laboratory,
St. Petersburg Pasteur Institute,
Russia

1

HBV & HCV Immunopathogenesis

Megha U. Lokhande, Joaquín Miquel, Selma Benito and Juan-R Larrubia
Translational Hepatology Unit, Guadalajara University Hospital, University of Alcalá
Spain

1. Introduction

Hepatitis B and C (HBV&HCV) viruses are two hepatotropic non-cytopathic viruses able to evade immune system efficiently as mechanism to persist in infected hosts. To fight against a viral infection the host displays two kinds of immune responses: the innate and adptive responses. The innate response is the first immunological barrier and it is essential in cytopathic viruses. This response limits viral spreading but also acts as adaptive response activator through antigen presentation to viral specific cells. Adaptive response is the second line in the immunological defense. It plays a major role in non-cytopathic viral infections because this type of viruses behaves as an intracellular parasite and they remain occult to the innate system.

1.1 General features of Innate Immune response

The liver is a unique anatomical and immunological site in which antigens-rich blood from the gastrointestinal tract is passed through a network of sinusoids and scanned by antigen-presenting cells and lymphocytes. It is selectively enriched in macrophages (Kupffer cells), natural killer cells (NK) and natural killer T cells (NKT) which are key components of the innate immune system (Racanelli & Rehermann, 2006).
Innate immunity generally plays a role immediately after infection to limit the spread of the pathogen and to activate the adaptive immune response (Guidotti & Chisari, 2006). Complex interplay between innate and adaptive immunity is the key for the resolution of acute infections. Innate response is induced after host recognition of common molecular patterns expressed by viruses, immediately after primoinfection, and providing a mandatory environment for triggering efficient adaptive immune responses. During hide and seek game of virus and host, one or more viral products get exposed and recognized by early immune response. This starts anti-viral control through direct cytopathic mechanisms (Koyama *et al.*, 1998), antiviral effect by producing IFN type I (IFN-alpha/beta) by infected cells (Samuel, 2001), and activation of the cellular component of the innate immune system as natural killer (NK) cells and natural killer T (NKT) cells (Biron *et al.*, 1999).
Production of type I IFNs can be triggered directly by virus replication through cellular mechanisms that detect the presence of viral RNA or DNA (Alexopoulou *et al.*, 2001), while NK cells are activated by the recognition of stress-induced molecules and/or the modulation of the quantity of major histocompatibility complex (MHC) class I molecules on the surface of infected cells (Moretta *et al.*, 2005).

NK and NKT cells can be rapidly recruited to the site of virus infection and have the potential to recognize infected cells before MHC class I expression is significantly induced on the cell surface. Activated NK and NKT cells may participate in disease pathogenesis directly, by killing infected cells, and indirectly, by producing soluble factors that have antiviral activity, recruiting inflammatory cells into the infected tissue and shaping the adaptive immune response (Biron *et al.*, 1999).

1.2 General features of adaptive immune response

Non-cytopathic viruses behave as intracellular parasites which are hidden to the immune system. They are not usually highly infectious but produce long-lasting diseases that allow them to spread the infection along the time. The host-virus relationship is a dynamic process in which the virus tries to decrease its visibility, whereas the host attempts to prevent and eradicate infection with minimal collateral damage to itself (Nowak & Bangham, 1996).

To control non-cytopathic viral infections, it is necessary the activation of the adaptive immune system, and especially the cellular immune response. Naïve specific CD4+ and CD8+ T cells are primed by dendritic cells in the lymph nodes. Once these cells become activated, they change the phenotype into effector cells and migrate to the infected tissue, attracted by the chemokines produced by the parenchymal cells. Primed specific CD4+ cells are essential to allow the adequate activation of specific cytotoxic T cells by secretion of Th1 cytokines (Larrubia *et al.*, 2009a). This is very important because specific cytotoxic T lymphocytes play a major role in spontaneous infection resolution. These cells are able to recognize the infected cells and to destroy them by cytolytic mechanisms, but they also produce type-1 cytokines that eliminate the virus without producing tissue damage (Fig.-1).

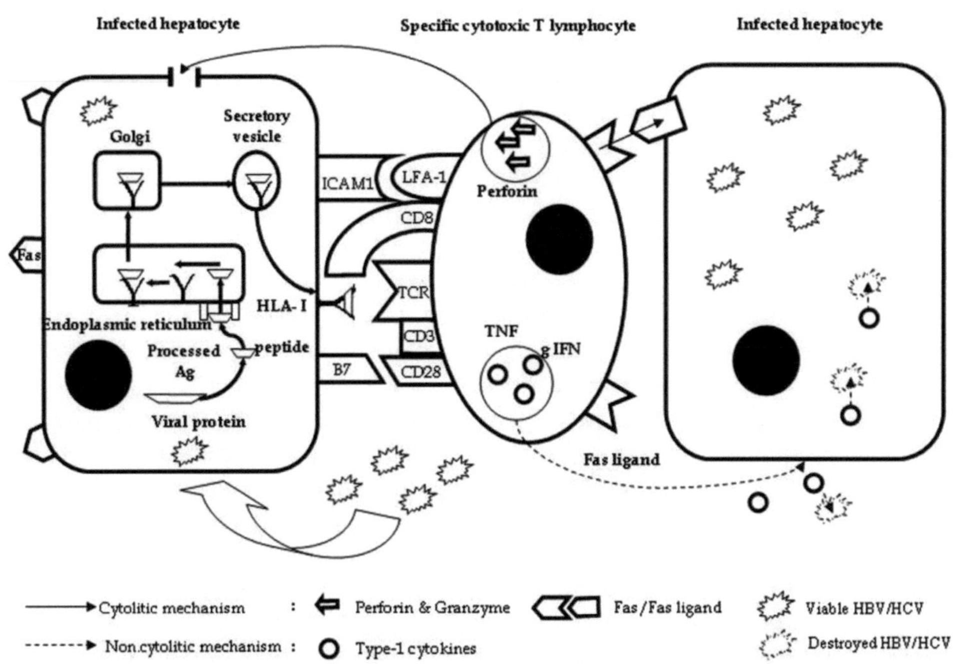

Fig. 1. Cytolitic and non-cytolitic mechanisms to destroy hepatotropic viruses by specific cytotoxic T cells

Both CD4+ and CD8+ cell activation depends on the engagement between T cell receptor and the MHC molecule/epitope complex plus the interaction between co-stimulatory molecules and their ligands (Choudhuri *et al.*, 2005). When these cells have finished their effector task, they express negative co-stimulatory molecules and pro-apoptotic factors to switch-off their activity, and a subsequent constriction in the specific T cell population is produced. After this event, a memory T cell population is maintained for decades to respond faster to a new infection, and in certain cases to keep under control viral occult infection (Appay *et al.*, 2008).

In this chapter the specific features of the immune response against two hepatotropic non-cytopathic viruses (HBV&HCV) able to induce a persistent infection in human are reviewed.

2. HBV immunopathogenesis

HBV is an enveloped incomplete circular double strand DNA virus. This virus is spread around the world and more than 2 billion people have markers of current or past HBV infection, developing chronic infection in approximately 350 million people. Approximately a quarter of persistent infection patients will develop terminal liver disease. The infection is acquired by parenteral, vertical and sexual transmission, and although there is an efficient vaccine, this infection is still an overwhelming health problem, especially in developing countries. Natural HBV control is based on a competent immune response but this is not obtained in 5-10% of infected adults and up to 95% of newborns from HBeAg-positive mothers (Liaw *et al*, 2010). Currently, there are different effective treatments able to control HBV replication but they are not very efficient in inducing either HBeAg or HB surface (HBsAg) Ag seroconversion (Perrillo *et al*, 2010). For this reason, it is interesting to understand the HBV immunopathogenesis to develop immunomodulatory strategies to restore an efficient anti-HBV immunoresponse.

2.1 Life cycle of HBV

Hepatitis B virus (HBV) is not directly cytopathic for the hepatocyte. During the early phase of HBV (before virus-specific T cells enter into the liver), there is no histological or biochemical evidence of hepatocyte damage (Guidotti *et al.*, 1999). Moreover, when cellular immune responses are deficient or pharmacologically suppressed, HBV can replicate at high levels in the liver in the absence of detectable pathological consequences (Ferrari *et al.*, 2003; Wieland *et al.*, 2000). These results suggest that hepatocyte damage during HBV infection is an immune-mediated event. Therefore, this virus is capable to enter, replicate and spread in human hepatocytes without causing any direct damage.

HBV is able to attach to the hepatocyte in a non-cell-type specific manner through cell-associated heparan sulphate proteoglycans. Later, the virus binds irreversibly to an unknown hepatocyte-specific preS1 receptor. After that, two different entry pathways have been proposed: endocytosis and fusion. Finally, the cytoplasmic release of the viral nucleocapsid, containing the relaxed circular partially double stranded DNA (rcDNA), is performed. Then, the nucleocapsid with the rcDNA is transported to the host cell nucleus (Kann *et al.*, 2007). Once rcDNA enters into the nucleus is repaired to complete the double strand DNA to produce the covalently closed circular DNA (cccDNA). The cccDNA stays stable in the hepatocyte nucleus for decades, and it is organized as chromatin like structure (minichromosome) (Levrero *et al.*, 2009). The cccDNA utilizes the cellular transcriptional machinery to produce all viral RNAs necessary for protein synthesis and viral replication.

From an immunological point of view, the cccDNA is extremely important since it will persist in most of the hepatocytes and it is not possible for the immune system to destroy it. For this reason, even if the immune response is able to control HBV infection, it does not mean HBV eradication because cccDNA persists as occult HBV infection in the hepatocytes (Larrubia, 2011; Rehermann *et al.*, 1996). From the pregenomic HBV RNA reverse transcription is performed by HBV DNA polymerase. This new HBV DNA can be either re-imported into the nucleus to form additional cccDNA molecules or can be enveloped with HBV translated proteins for secretion (Urban *et al.*, 2010).

2.2 HBV acute infection

2.2.1 Innate immune response during acute HBV infection

During HBV primo-infection, replication can be efficiently limited by type I IFNs (Wieland *et al.*, 2000; McClary *et al.*, 2000). Nevertheless, data on acutely infected chimpanzees have shown a lack of detection of genes associated to innate response in the liver during the entry and expansion phase of HBV (Wieland *et al.*, 2004). During this phase, HBV can replicate unchecked to extremely high levels. It has been proposed that, because HBV replicates within nucleocapsid particles, viral replicative intermediates of single-stranded RNA or viral DNA, which are strong activators of type I IFN genes, are protected from cellular recognition (Wieland & Chisari, 2005).

Such early events are difficult to analyze during natural infection in humans, because HBV-infected patients are mainly detected after clinical hepatitis, which occur 10-12 weeks after infection. Nevertheless, it is interesting to note that the lack of early symptoms (such as fever and malaise) in HBV-infected patients, typical of other human viral infections, constitutes an indirect evidence of the defective type-I IFN production during the early phases of HBV infection.

In a cohort of patients, sampled in the pre-clinical phase and followed up to infection resolution, serum concentrations of IFN-alpha remained barely detectable during the early incubation phase and throughout the peak of viral replication and subsequent viral load reduction. Circulating IFN-alpha levels in patients with acute HBV infection at the time of peak of viremia were no significantly greater than at the time of infection resolution. Similarly, IFN-kappa and IL-15, which are important for induction of NK effector function, were not induced during the peak of viremia (Dunn *et al.*, 2009).

Consequently, HBV can be considered as a "stealth virus", capable of sneaking through the front line of host defenses. It is possible that this situation of immune suppression might be activated by HBV replication. IL-10 is a potent immunosuppressive cytokine that can inhibit both innate and adaptive immunity. In fact, a close correlation between circulating IL-10 and HBV-DNA levels have been observed. IL-10 increased early in the course of infection, in parallel with the rapid increase in HBV viral load and antigenaemia and before the onset of inflammation. Moreover, the reduction of IL-10 coincided with either the termination of viremia or with HBeAg seroconversion. Consequently, there may be an active suppression of NK responses mediated for IL-10. In further support of this, addition of exogenous IL-10 during in-vitro experiments was able to suppress NK cell IFN-gamma production which was recovered upon blocking IL-10 and its receptor (Dunn *et al.*, 2009).

Although no induction of type-I interferon is observed, within hours after HBV infection, there is a transient release of IL-6 and other proinflammatory cytokines (IL-8, tumour necrosis factor (TNF) alfa, IL-1B). The IL-6 released was shown to control HBV gene transcription and replication in hepatocytes shortly after infection, ensuring an early control of virus replication, thereby limiting the activation of the adaptive immune response and preventing death of the HBV-infected hepatocytes in the early phases of infection (Hosel *et al.*, 2009). The production of IL-6 and other cytokines seems transient after HBV infection. Interestingly, HBV replication tends to increase 3-4 days after infection, when IL-6 level has returned to baseline. This may suggest that the virus actively counteracts the action of IL-6, like occurs during the human cytomegalovirus infection (Gealy *et al.*, 2005).

However, a role for the innate immune response in the control of early HBV replication should not be dismissed. A study performed in woodchucks (Guy *et al.*, 2008) observed a NK and NKT cell response within hours after inoculation with a liver-pathogenic dose of woodchuck hepatitis virus. These immune responses were at least partially capable of limiting viral propagation but were not followed by a prompt adaptive T cell response, which was delayed for 4-5weeks. Chimpanzees able to control the virus show a typical acute phase of disease with a robust activation of IFN-gamma, and TNF-alpha (Guidotti *et al.*, 1999). It is possible that this initial host response to HBV is primarily sustained by NK and NKT cells, that are capable to inhibit HBV replication in-vivo (Kakimi *et al.*, 2000), as shown by the early development of NK and NKT responses in healthy blood donors who became hepatitis B surface antigen and HBV DNA positive (Fisicaro *et al.*, 2009). Also, an early activation of NK and NKT cells in a woodchuck model of acute hepatitis B infection has been shown. In this model NK and NKT cells induced a transient, but significant reduction of virus replication (Guy *et al.*, 2008).

In human, a study performed in two seronegative blood donors who became positive for HBsAg and HBV DNA, who were monitored throughout very early stages of infection, demonstrated that the human innate immune system is indeed capable of sensing HBV early after infection and of triggering a NK/NKT cell response to contain HBV infection and to allow a timely induction of adaptive response (Fisicaro *et al.*, 2009).

Therefore, rather than being silent, hepadnaviruses may be efficient at counteracting the actions of the innate immune system early after infection. There is a growing body of evidence suggesting that HBV could inhibit innate responses by regulating the expression of Toll-like receptors (TLRs), which are major sensors of viral infection in immune-specialized and non-specialized cells (Barton, 2007). HBV is able to suppress toll-like receptor-mediated innate immune response in murine parenchymal and non-parenchymal liver cells (Wu *et al.*, 2009). Indeed, the expression of TLR1, TLR2, TLR4 and TLR6 is significantly lower in peripheral blood mononuclear cells (PBMC) and hepatocytes from chronic hepatitis B (CHB) patients (Chen *et al.*, 2008). Furthermore, flow cytometric analysis has shown that the expression of TLR2 in PBMC, from CHB patients is significantly decreased. TLR2 expression on PBMC has been correlated with the HBsAg plasma levels (Riordan *et al.*, 2006) and HBeAg protein (Visvanathan *et al.*, 2007). Recently, an immunomodulatory role of HBeAg on innate immune signal transduction pathways, via interaction and targeting of TLR-mediated signalling pathways, has also been shown (Lang *et al*,.2011).

Moreover, dendritic cells (DC) exhibit functional impairment in hepatitis B virus carriers. Plasmocytoid (p)-DC are the major type-I interferon producing cells and sensors of viral infections because they express both TLR7 and TLR9 that respectively recognize, even in absence of viral replication, single-stranded RNA and unmethylated cytosine-guanosine dinucleotide motifs (Fitzgerald-Bocarsly *et al.*, 2008). A recent study reported that, in CHB patients, there was a reduction of TLR-9 expressions in pCDs, which correlates with an impaired IFN-alpha production by these cells (Xie *et al.*, 2009).

Altogether, these data suggest that HBV infection can alter innate immune responses, triggered by both specialized cells and hepatocytes, through down-regulating functional expression of TLR. Currently, whether HBV is a stealth virus for the innate immune response or is able to block it efficiently is a matter of debate.

2.2.2 Adaptive response during acute HBV infection

Despite of the lack of proper innate response activation, this does not affect to adaptive response during HBV primo-infection. HBV-specific T cell response appears soon after the exponential HBV replication phase (Webster *et al.*, 2000). Both, CD4+ and CD8+ specific responses are present and they are polyclonal, vigorous and multi-specific, when the viral control is obtained, while these responses are impaired when the infection progresses over chronicity (Maini *et al.*, 1999). HBV control is achieved through the labor of HBV-specific CD8+ T cells. These cells are able to recognize infected hepatocytes and to destroy them by apoptosis, but also they produce type-I cytokines, such as gamma-interferon and TNF-alpha, which are capable of non-cytopathic HBV clearing (Ferrari *et al.*, 2003; Guidotti & Chisari, 2001). This response to become fully activated needs the adequate stimulation by professional antigen presenting cells and the correct regulation by specific CD4+ cells. HBV-specific CD8+ T cells are responsible of HBV control, but they also initiate a minor liver damage. In fact, most HBV DNA is eliminated by non-cytolitic pathways before amino-transferases elevation is detected. Nevertheless, the secreted IFN-gamma by these cells, in addition to the chemokines produced by infected hepatocytes, attracts non-specific mononuclear cells and polymorphonuclear cells, which are responsible of liver damage amplification (Guidotti & Chisari, 2006). This phenomenon is also acting in the pathogenesis of chronic disease. Specifically, during persistent infection, the HBV specific response is impaired and unable to control the infection, but the hepatocytes continue secreting chemokines to attract effector T cells. However, non-specific inflammatory cells are also attracted and they are the cause of the low grade of persistent liver damage (Bertoletti & Maini, 2000).

During the acute phase of infection, antibodies (Ab) against HBsAg, HBeAg and core (HBc) Ag are produced by activated B cells. HBsAb and HBeAb production is T helper dependent, while HBcAb secretion is dependent and non-dependent from T helper action (Milich & Chisari, 1982). HBs antibodies are produced very early after infection, but they are not detected because they generate complexes with circulating antigens, and therefore they are not detected until the virus is controlled. HBs antibodies prevent viral spreading from one to another hepatocyte and also block circulating HBV. The detection of these antibodies means HBV control and confers natural immunity against re-infection. Observation of HBsAb occurs when HBV is controlled by immune system, and these are neutralizing Abs that will avoid HBV re-infection in case of a new encounter with the virus. HBc Abs are not neutralizing and they indicate HBV contact. When HBc IgM subtype is positive it means acute infection or HBV flare-up during chronic infection. HBe Abs appear before HBs Abs during acute HBV recovery and also when chronic patients shift from a replicative to a non-replicative phase. Moreover, HBe Abs are also present during the HBV chronic replicative phase, when the infecting virus displays a pre-core mutation that avoids HBe Ag production (Maruyama *et al.*, 1994; Milich & Liang, 2003).

During adulthood, most of acute HBV infected cases recover and develop natural immunity due to the combination of a polyclonal, vigorous and multispecific cytotoxic and helper response (Guidotti & Chisari, 2006). After a self-limited infection, a T cell response constriction is observed and a central memory T cell population is generated. In these cases, a long-lasting protective T cell response is developed. These cells keep under control the intrahepatic HBV traces for decades. In fact, in HBV recovered patients it is possible to demonstrate a T1 orientated multispecific cytotoxic and helper response, decades after primo-infection, and those responses are associated with the observation of HBV DNA in sera or PBMC using ultra-sensitive PCR techniques. These data show that HBV recovery does not mean HBV eradication, since despite of clinical recovery it is possible to demonstrate HBV viral traces that are maintained under control due to the adaptive memory immune response (Larrubia, 2011; Penna *et al.*, 1996; Rehermann *et al.*, 1996).

2.3 HBV chronic infection

Around 5-10% of HBV primoinfection progresses to chronicity in adult infection, while it reaches 95% of newborns from HBeAg-positive mothers and approximately 50% during childhood infection (Liaw *et al.*, 2010). The development of a persistent HBV infection is based on a failure of HBV-specific response due to the induction of an anergic and pro-apoptotic status on this response because of the high viral pressure (Maini *et al.*, 2000a; Webster *et al.*, 2004). Several mechanisms have been involved in the impairment of specific T cell response. Specific T cells behave as anergic cells with progressive impairment of type-1 cytokine production, such as IL-2, IFN-gamma and TNF-alpha. The cytotoxic T cells are neither able to proliferate nor to kill infected hepatocytes after antigen encounter. Nevertheless, cytokines and chemokines produced in the infected liver are able to attract a non-specific inflammatory population causing the persistent liver damage. Several mechanisms are used by HBV to induce this anergic status, which will end-up in a pro-apoptotic situation that could cause specific T cell deletion. Persistent high HBs antigenemia, massive production of defective viral particles and the toleraising liver environment induces an anergic condition on T cells. In fact, HBV infected liver is depleted in tryptophan and there is an accumulation in its toxic metabolite (IDO) which is able to induce immunotolerance (Larrea *et al.*, 2007). Also, arginase I activity is increased during HBV infection provoking an arginine depletion on T cells which causes a CD3ζ down-regulation. The effect of CD3ζ lower expression translates into IL-2 production impairment by HBV-specific CD8+ cells (Das *et al.*, 2008). Interestingly, in the HBV infected liver is increased the secretion of immunosuppressive cytokines. IL-10 is produced by dendritic cells and Kupffer cells while transforming growth factor-beta (TGF-β) is secreted by stellate cells. The level of these cytokines correlates with HBV disease activity during chronic and acute infection (Dunn *et al.*, 2009). Other escape mechanisms involve TRAIL-mediated deletion of HBV-specific CD8+ cells by NK cells (Dunn *et al.*, 2007). Moreover, regulatory T cells can cause HBV-specific T cell activity suppression (Furuichi *et al.*, 2005). On the other hand, persistent HBV infection favors the up-regulation of pro-apoptotic molecule Bim. This molecule mediates premature HBV specific cytotoxic T cell death following intrahepatic antigen presentation (Lopes *et al.*, 2008). Another common mechanism, induced by HBV to evade immune system, is the induction of negative co-stimulatory molecules such as CTLA-4, PD-1, Tim3 and Lag3. Excessive co-inhibitory signals drive T cell exhaustion during chronic HBV-infection (Maini & Schurich, 2010). Finally, HBV is also able to evade specific immune response by developing escape mutation at cytotoxic and helper immunodominant epitopes (Maini *et al.*, 2000b).

2.3.1 Adaptive response during chronic HBV infection

Chronic evolving infection is characterized by several progressive phases with different adaptive response features. The first stage is called immunotolerant phase. This is typical for countries with high rates of mother to child HBV transmission, but it is not seen in Western countries, where this route of transmission is not common. During this phase, HBV viral load is extremely high, but the liver damage and the anti-HBV immune response are absent. Several studies from D. Milich group, in HBe+ transgenic mice, have shown that the lack of HBV-specific immune response is due to some properties of HBeAg. This viral protein is able to cross the placenta to reach the offsprings thymus, where this is considered a self-antigen, eliciting HBe/HBc Ag-specific T helper cell tolerance in uterus (Milich *et al.*, 1990). Moreover, during this phase, high HBV viral load inhibits adaptive immune response. In fact, frequency and function of HBV-specific T cells is inversely correlated with HBV viral load (Boni *et al.*, 2007; Webster *et al.*, 2004) (Fig.-2). In the natural history of chronic HBV infection, this phase is followed by the immuno-clearance stage. This is the common starting point in persistent infection in Western countries. This phase is characterized by viral replication and liver damage fluctuations. Even though the specific immune response is quite inefficient, it is still able to obtain certain HBV control. During this phase, HBeAg seroconversion and HBV pre-core mutant selection is possible. HBe seroconversion allows the change to another HBV infection phase with a higher viral control and lower liver damage. HBe seroconversion is faster in individuals with certain polymorphisms at IL-10 and IL-12 genes. In these cases, high levels of IL-10 and IL-12 are observed and they are a predictor of spontaneous HBe seroconversion (Wu *et al.*, 2010). Another typical feature of the immuno-clearance phase is the presence of HBV exacerbations, characterized by HBeAg level increase followed by transaminase level raise. The HBeAg level increase induces an activation of HBc/HBe specific response activation, after this a decrease in HBeAg and transminase level is observed, followed by a specific T cell response constriction. This data show that HBV-specific T cell activation due to HBeAg level is causing acute exacerbations in HBeAg+ chronic patients (Frelin *et al.*, 2009). This phenomenon can lead to liver damage generation, HBe seroconversion and pre-core mutant selection. During these HBV acute exacerbations, HBV-specific cytotoxic T cells destroy wild-type HBV infected hepatocyte producing liver damage. Moreover, if along this stage HBV pre-core mutants emerge, these cytotoxic T cells can select them, since the infected hepatocytes with these variants are not recognized properly by cytotoxic T cells. In fact, liver infected cells by the wild type virus are eliminated more efficiently by specific cytotoxic T cells than cells infected by the pre-core mutant. This is because wild-type infected cells presenting HBc and HBe epitopes are better targets for cytotoxic T cells than cells infected by HBV pre-core mutant expressing only core epitopes (Frelin *et al.*, 2009). This situation leads to HBe antigen negative form of chronic hepatitis B with persistent liver damage, which is different to the wild-type HBe seroconversion where the infection can be consider inactive. This last one is the third phase of the chronic HBV natural history which is called low or non replicative phase, and corresponds to the clinical inactive carrier state. In this stage viral load and liver damage is very low. During this phase HBV-specific T cell responses are present and are quite efficient despite lack of liver damage. These cells are very competent in controlling infected hepatocytes, preventing HBV spreading and the development of liver infiltration by non-specific inflammatory cells, which are the cause of persistent liver damage during chronic active hepatitis B. Therefore, it is considered that during the low/non-replicative phase HBV is under a partial control by HBV-specific response (Maini *et al.*, 2000a). At this stage, it is possible to observe HBV reactivation associated with hepatitis flares, mainly in the case of infection by HBV pre-core mutants. This last phase of HBV natural history is called reactivation phase. The immunological causes of these reactivations are not very well known yet. During these hepatitis flares is not possible to demonstrate the presence of HBV-specific T cell reactivity, but it is observed NK cell activation which correlates with the degree of liver damage (Dunn *et al.*, 2007). Therefore, in this last step of chronic HBV natural history, the innate response could be involved.

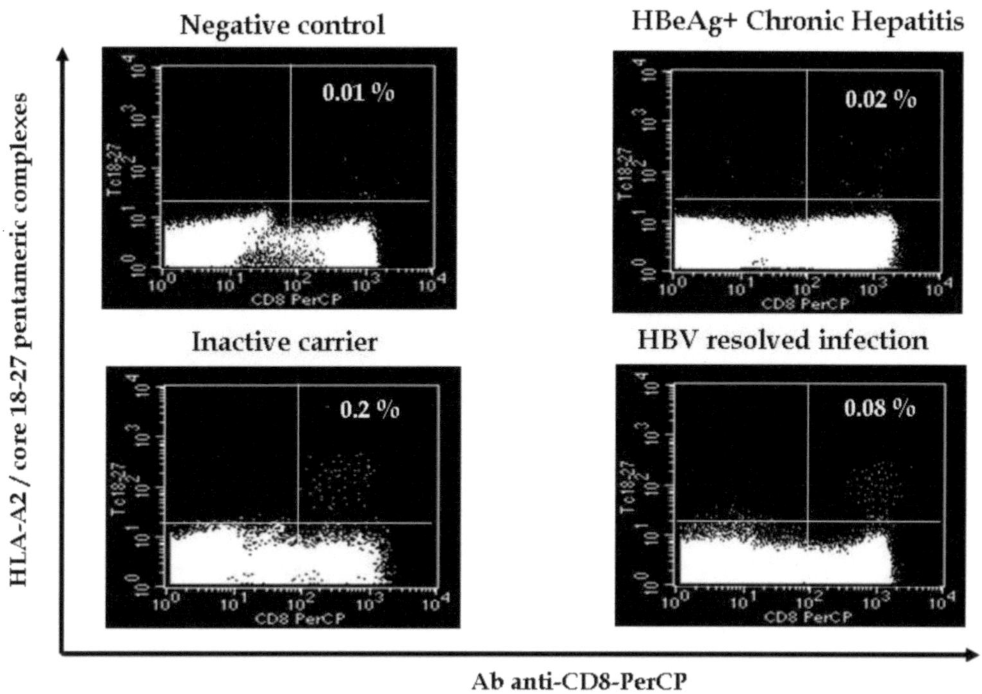

Fig. 2. FACS® dot-plots from peripheral blood mononuclear cells of HBV infected patients with different HBV control stained directly ex-vivo with Ab against CD8 plus multimeric HLA-A2/core 18-27 complexes. A negative correlation between viral control and frequency of HBV-sepcific CD8+ cells is observed. Figures in the upper right quadrant show the frequency of HBV-specific CD8+ cells out of total CD8 population.

In summary, HBV is not ever completely eliminated from the infected host, but there is a gradient of control according to the functional efficiency of HBV-specific response. In patients with HBV natural immunity, they present a HBV occult infection with a very efficient control by CD4+ and CD8+ specific HBV T cells. This immune control is partial in patients in the inactive carrier state and completely inefficient in cases with chronic active hepatitis (Boni *et al.*, 2007; Maini *et al.*, 2000a; Zerbini *et al.*, 2008). Strategies directed to restore anti-HBV adaptive response could help in the permanent infection control.

3. HCV immunopathogenesis

The hepatitis C virus (HCV) is an enveloped; positive stranded RNA virus and represents the Hepacivirus genus in the Flaviviridae family. It has been estimated that more than 170 million people are infected with HCV, since clinical identification and molecular cloning of HCV in late 1980s. This virus is spread by contact with infected blood and body fluids. Approximately 80% of infections succeed in establishing a chronic infection with the potential for developing severe liver diseases such as cirrhosis and hepatocellular carcinoma (HCC) (Lavanchy, 2009; Tsukuma *et al.*, 1993).

No effective vaccine against HCV is available till date. Current standard-of-care therapy for HCV infection as peg-interferon-alpha and ribavirin (Pawlotsky, 2004), has limited efficacy, in particular against the genotype 1 virus (Fried *et al.*, 2002; Manns *et al.*, 2001). An extended search for new therapy is progressing, already passed for marketing authorization of the protease-inhibitors (Poordad *et al*, 2011). A major concern with new therapy is rapid development of drug-resistant viral mutants. Due to the failure or side effect of the treatment, stepping forward for understanding the immunopathogenesis of HCV infection is essential in the development of a therapeutic vaccine and immunomodulatory treatments for chronic infections.

Due to the lack of adequate cell culture systems, HCV studies have been slowed down for a long time, but continuous progress in the last few years it has overcome this obstacle. In-vivo model to study the biology of HCV have been significantly restricted due to the limited experimental availability of chimapanzees, the primary model for HCV (Alter *et al.*, 1978; Bukh, 2004), and difficulties encountered in reproducing true infection in small animals. Two breakthroughs has been an important contribution to the field: firstly, subgenomic replicons (i.e. without structural genes) (Blight *et al.*, 2000; Blight *et al.*, 2003; Lohmann *et al.*, 1999), which are highly permissive for HCV replication (Blight *et al.*, 2002) and secondly, HCV complete replication in cell culture (Lindenbach *et al.*, 2005; Wakita *et al.*, 2005; Zhong *et al.*, 2005). However, it has long been recognized that these models are complicated by the particularly high error rate of the HCV RNA replicase (Rong *et al.*, 2010).

It is widely accepted that immune-mediated host-virus interactions are responsible for the outcome of HCV and pathogenesis of further severe diseases. In this chapter, it is covered how virus evades primary defense mechanisms. Finally, adaptive immune response escape mechanisms induced by HCV to become persistent are also analyzed. To be familiar with pathogenesis of HCV infection, a brief outline of HCV life cycle is provided below.

3.1 Life cycle of HCV

The development of HCV replicons (Blight *et al.*, 2000; Blight *et al.*, 2003; Ikeda *et al.*, 2002; Lohmann *et al.*, 1999), HCV pseudotyped particles (HCVpp) (Bartosch *et al.*, 2003a) and most recently the infectious HCV cell culture system (Lindenbach *et al.*, 2005; Wakita *et al.*, 2005; Zhong *et al.*, 2005) have advanced our understanding of the viral life cycle. Hepatocytes are the primary site of HCV infections. HCV life cycle begins with binding of the virus to cell surface receptors. The putative receptors, the tetraspanin protein CD81 (Bartosch *et al.*, 2003a; Hsu *et al.*, 2003; Pileri *et al.*, 1998; Wunschmann *et al.*, 2000), the scavenger receptor class B member I (SR-B1) (Bartosch *et al.*, 2003a; Grove *et al.*, 2007; Kapadia *et al.*, 2007; Scarselli *et al.*, 2002) and the tight junction proteins claudin-1 (Evans *et al.*, 2007) and occluding, (Benedicto *et al.*, 2009; Liu *et al.*, 2009; Ploss *et al.*, 2009) have all been shown to enable HCV entry. In addition, the low-density lipoprotein receptor (Agnello *et al.*, 1999;

Molina *et al.*, 2007; Monazahian *et al.*, 1999; Wunschmann *et al.*, 2000), asialoglycoprotein receptor (Saunier *et al.*, 2003), and glycosaminoglycans (heparin sulfate) are also involved, but their exact roles have not been determined. By clathrinmediated endocytosis (Blanchard *et al.*, 2006; Meertens *et al.*, 2006), HCV enters the cell. The virus undergoes an uncoating process by fusion between the viral envelope and endosomal membrane in the acidified endosomal compartment (Bartosch *et al.*, 2003b; Haid *et al.*, 2009; Hsu *et al.*, 2003; Koutsoudakis *et al.*, 2006; Lavillette *et al.*, 2006; Tscherne *et al.*, 2006) via E1/E2-mediated class II fusion (Garry & Dash, 2003; Lavillette *et al.*, 2007), to expose the viral genomic RNA to host-cell machinery. About ~9.6 kb viral RNA genome is released into the host cell cytoplasm, to serve as template for the translation of the viral proteins. IRES-mediated translation of the HCV genome produces a single ~3,000 amino-acid polyprotein (Moradpour *et al.*, 2004), which is processed by cellular and viral proteases into at least 10 different protein products. These products include the structural proteins, which form the viral particle (the virus core and the envelope proteins E1 and E2), and the nonstructural proteins P7, NS3, NS4A, NS4B, NS5A and NS5B (Guidotti & Chisari, 2006). Viral replication is driven by minus strand intermediate. HCV double stranded RNA (dsRNA) is freely exposed in the cytoplasm of infected cell (Moradpour *et al.*, 2004), which is recognizable for host innate immune system. Nucleocapsid is formed by assembling capsid proteins and genomic RNA and bud through intracellular membranes into cytoplasmic vesicles. Finally, by secretory pathway, mature enveloped virions release from the cell.

3.2 Innate immune response during acute HCV infection

The first response to HCV protein is thought to be IFN-β production by infected hepatocytes, which are able to secrete type I IFN. The infected cells are sensed with pathogen associated molecular patterns (PAMP), Toll like receptor (TLR3) (Marie *et al.*, 1998) and retinoic acid-inducible gene I (RIG-I) (Bauer *et al.*, 2001; Sato *et al.*, 2000) by endosomal dsRNA and cytosolic dsRNA respectively, which is an essential intermediate in the HCV replication cycle, and thus, they may be important in the pathogenesis of hepatitis C (Saito *et al.*, 2008). RIG-I recruits IFN-β promoter stimulator protein 1 (IPS-1; also called CARD adaptor inducing IFN-β CARDIF), virus-induced signaling adapter (VISA), and mitochondrial antiviral signaling protein (MAVS) (Hoshino *et al.*, 2006; Meylan *et al.*, 2005; Xu *et al.*, 2005), after ATP-driven activity dependant on recognition of viral protein (Honda *et al.*, 2004). On other hand, TLR3 dimerization, due to leucine-rich repeats (Liu *et al.*, 1998), recruits the adapter protein, Toll–IL-1 receptor domain-containing adaptor inducing IFN-β (TRIF). Both processes result in downstream signaling, nuclear translocation of IFN regulatory factor 3 (IRF3) and leads to stimulation of the transcription of a set of genes including IFN-β (Kawai & Akira, 2008). Antiviral state, induced by secreted IFN β, gives an alert to uninfected cells by activation of effector molecules. Binding of IFN α-β to cognate receptor complex lead to the activation of JAK/STAT pathway, which results in the induction of IFN-stimulated genes (ISGs) and lead to enhance the IFN response (Rehermann, 2009) (Fig.- 3).

However, HCV has organized a number of countermeasures not only to inhibit the induction phase, but also interfere with the effector phase of the IFN system (Fig.- 3). It has been confirmed, in in-vitro studies, that HCV serine protease, NS3/4A is enable to cleave MAVS (Li *et al.*, 2005b), TRIF (Li *et al.*, 2005a), IPS-1 (Foy *et al.*, 2003) and oligomerization of MAVS, which is part of signaling process (Kawaguchi *et al.*, 2004; Li *et al.*, 2005a; Li *et al.*, 2005b; Marie *et al.*, 1998; Meylan *et al.*, 2005; Sakamoto *et al.*, 2000). Disruption of IRF-3 activation occurred by NS3 protein action (Liu *et al.*, 1999) and it has been shown with different cell lines in-vitro studies (Kawaguchi *et al.*, 2004; Marie *et al.*, 1998). Another key player, HCV core, when over expressed in cell culture, disturbs antiviral activity via interfering in JAK/STAT signaling and ISG expression by inhibition of STAT1 activation. Simultaneously it induces its degradation (Gale & Foy, 2005; Lin *et al.*, 2006) by induction of inhibitor of the JAK/STAT pathway SOCS3 (Bode *et al.*, 2003), protein phosphatase 2A (PP2A), which ultimately reduces the transcriptional activity of ISG factor 3 (ISGF3) (Heim *et al.*, 1999); and inhibition of ISGF3 interaction to IFN-stimulated response elements (Rehermann, 2009). HCV NS5A interferes with the function of ISGs by inhibiting 2'-5' oligoadenylate synthetase (2'-5' OAS) and leads to overall ISG expression impairment (Polyak *et al.*, 2001). Protein kinase R (PKR) can negatively regulate HCV replication noncytolytically in cell cultures (Kim *et al.*, 2004; Zhao *et al.*, 2004), which can interacts with HCV NS5A and lost its function. Interestingly, HCV E2 acts as distraction target to PKR (Taylor *et al.*, 1999). To sum up, the main targets of HCV proteins to evade immune response are interference with the induction of IFN synthesis, IFN- induced intracellular signaling and IFN-induced effector mechanisms (Fig.-3).

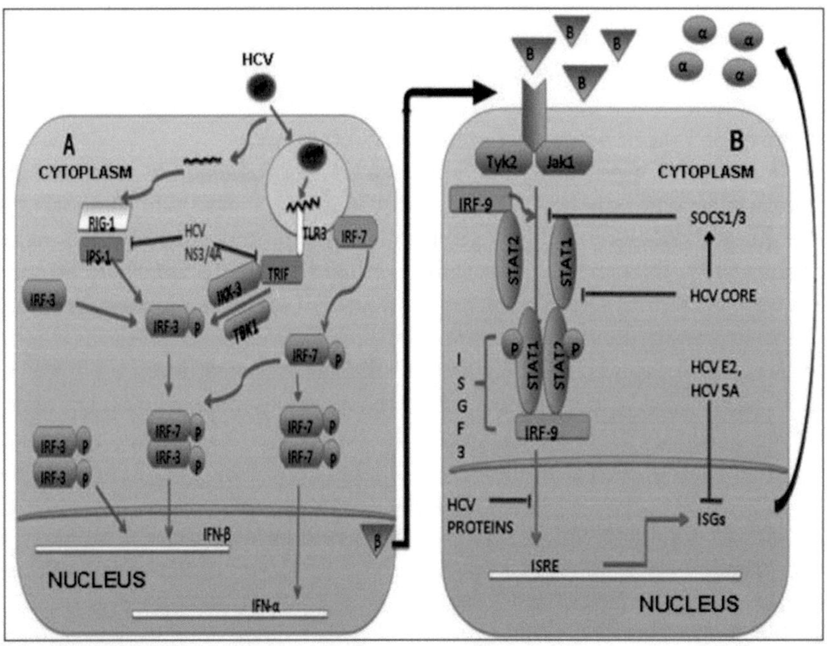

Fig. 3. Evasion of Innate immune response by HCV: (A) Interference in IFN synthesis: Blocking of TLR 3 and RIG-1 signalling respectively, by cleavage of the adaptor molecule TRIF and IPS-1 via HCV NS3/4A; (B) Interference in IFN-induced effector mechanisms: Binding of IFN β and its receptor with TYK2 and JAK1 kinase activation lead to form ISGF3 complex, where this complex interact with IFN stimulated response elements (ISREs) within the promoter and enhancer region of ISGs to induce ISGs (such as 2', 5' OAS, PKR, IRF7) production in nucleus. HCV core induce SOCS1/3, which is the inhibitor of the JAK/STAT pathway and inhibits STAT1 phosphorylation, which inhibits assembly of trimeric ISGFs complex. Function of ISGs is inhibited by HCVE2 and HCV NS3/4A.

Dendritic cells (DC) are professional antigen presenting cells with important functions in antiviral immunity through activation of adaptive immune responses. Type-I IFNs are also produced by pDCs, which derive from the lymphoid lineage. Although, production of IFN alpha/beta, in early phase of infection occurs after recognition of ssRNA and dsRNA by TLR7 and TLR9 respectively, the mechanism is still not clear (Albert *et al.*, 2008). The frequency of pDCs in the blood (Nakamoto *et al.*, 2008) and their production of IFN-α in HCV infection is reduced after in vitro stimulation (Bowen *et al.*, 2008). The possible mechanism has been demonstrated in in-vitro studies. First, HCV core and NS3 activate monocytes by TLR2 signaling to produce TNF-α (Izaguirre *et al.*, 2003), which in turn inhibits IFN-α production and induces pDC apoptosis (Bowen *et al.*, 2008). Second, HCV itself inhibits IFN-α production of pDCs (Diepolder *et al.*, 1995). However, other studies revealed regular response to TLR stimulation by circulating pDCs of chronically infected individuals (Decalf *et al.*, 2007; Longman *et al.*, 2005) and they have high levels of endogenous type I IFNs without immuno-dysfuction (Albert *et al.*, 2008). Although this defense mechanism is significant, the host rarely overcomes HCV infection, which suggests several other viral evasion mechanisms that are poorly or not understood yet.

Another group of DCs, myeloid DCs (mDCs) derive from the myeloid lineage (Lanzavecchia & Sallusto, 2001; Steinman *et al.*, 2003). Due to its tolerogenic and stimulatory role (Lanzavecchia & Sallusto, 2001; Steinman *et al.*, 2003), mDCs have been broadly studied in HCV infection. mDCs have not been observed to be decrease in peripheral blood or dysfunctional in HCV chronic infected individuals in in-vitro studies (Kanto *et al.*, 1999; Longman *et al.*, 2004). Nevertheless, HCV proteins can interact with monocytes/macrophages through TLR2, inducing the IL-10 production, which hampers IL-12 production by mDC and IFN-alpha by pDC, or they directly inhibit DC differentiation (Szabo & Dolganiuc, 2005). IL-12 cytokine production by mDC is decreased in HCV patients in response to stimuli like CD40 L or poly (I:C) (Anthony *et al.*, 2004), which can explain clearly the shift from Th1 to Th2 response in HCV patients. In-vitro studies indicates that DC expressing core and E1 proteins have lower stimulatory ability, which is associated to the lack of maturation after stimulation with TNF-alpha or CD40L (Sarobe *et al.*, 2003).

Other cells involved in the innate response are the NK cells. Functions of these cells include generating a cytotoxic response, regulatory cytokines production and control on DC maturation and amplitude of DC response, which may deeply impact on type of down-stream adaptive immune responses. Response to HCV infection by NK cell is direct apoptosis induction of infected cells with production of antiviral cytokines (Golden-Mason & Rosen, 2006; Lodoen & Lanier, 2006). Moreover, NK cell depletion or dysfunction favor HCV persistence (Golden-Mason *et al.*, 2008). The role of interactions between HLA class I and killer cell–Ig-like receptors (KIR) during HCV infection has been shown. KIR can regulate NK cell activities. However puzzling contradictions for this topic in different studies have been revealed (Montes-Cano *et al.*, 2005; Paladino *et al.*, 2007; Rauch *et al.*, 2007). The importance of NK cells in the resolution of HCV infection is illustrated by the influence of genetic polymorphisms of KIR and their HLA ligands on the outcome of HCV infection, which was dependent on a homozygous HLA class I ligand background (Khakoo *et al.*, 2004; Knapp *et al.*, 2010; Stegmann *et al.*, 2010). There is need to focus on clear understanding of functional and molecular HLA-KIR interactions to know about the possible way for NK cell-mediated protection in animal models of HCV infection.

However, an increased proportion of NK cells expressing activating receptors, enhanced cytotoxicity and defective cytokine production have revealed in chronic HCV infection (Oliviero *et al.*, 2009). Megan et al revealed that IL28A cytokine could significantly inhibit IFN-γ production lead to NK cell inactivation (Ahlenstiel *et al.*, 2010), which would be important to attenuate chronically activated NK cells. Consequently, the analysis of functional scene between NK cells and type 3 IFN in the immune response to virus will be required to understand the role of the NK in disease progression during HCV infection.

3.3 Adaptive immune response

The second barrier to control HCV infection is the adaptive immunity. This response has two arms to fight against pathogens; humoral and cellular immune response. Humoral immune response, that means neutralizing and non-neutralizing antibodies can endorse antiviral activity and pathogenesis (Guidotti & Chisari, 2006). Cellular immune response shows antiviral immunity by means of virus specific CD8 cytotoxic T lymphocytes (CTLs) and CD4 T helper cells, which play key effector and regulatory roles respectively. These T cells take part in viral pathogenesis of HCV by direct killing of infected cells or producing soluble factors able to clear the virus in a non-cytolytic manner, but also can lead to HCV pathogenic events, favoring direct liver damage and attracting non-specific inflammatory cells to perpetuate the liver inflammation (Guidotti & Chisari, 2006).

3.3.1 Humoral immune response

Neutralizing antibodies (nAbs) generally play a critical role for controlling initial viremia and protecting from re-infection in viral infections. However, the role of the humoral immune response in the clearance of HCV infection has been in the dark for a long time due to difficulties to determine relative role of antibodies to neutralize HCV. It can exclusively be evaluated by relevant model systems. It is thought that HCV clearance could occur in the absence of nAbs. If they are present alone, these Abs are inadequate to eradicate HCV in most of the cases in early studies (Dustin & Rice, 2007; Lechner *et al.*, 2000a; Lechner *et al.*, 2000b; Logvinoff *et al.*, 2004; Thimme *et al.*, 2002).

It has been proved that HCV specific T cells may compensate for lack of neutralizing antibodies to obtain HCV clearance (Semmo *et al.*, 2006). However, due to the development of novel model systems (Bartosch *et al.*, 2003a; Baumert *et al.*, 1998; Lindenbach *et al.*, 2005; Wakita *et al.*, 2005; Zhong *et al.*, 2005), it is possible to focus on HCV entry into host cells and neutralization process which demonstrated that nAbs are induced by patients who subsequently control (Lavillette *et al.*, 2005) or resolve (Pestka *et al.*, 2007) viral infection in the early phase of infection and contrary in chronic infection. This suggests that a strong, early, broad nAbs response may contribute to resolution of HCV in the acute phase of infection while delayed induction of nAbs may contribute to development of chronic HCV infection.

Instead of the rapid, vigorous and multi-specific antiviral host immune responses, chronic patients have been shown to develop a delayed and inefficient neutralizing antibody response (Pestka *et al.*, 2007) due to HCV escape mechanism (Zeisel *et al.*, 2008). Recent studies evident that entry of HCV can be hampered or modulated by nAbs of chronic HCV patients (Gal-Tanamy *et al.*, 2008; Haberstroh *et al.*, 2008; Keck *et al.*, 2009), while it is controversial in cell culture study (Grove *et al.*, 2008). In addition, although nAbs are incapable to clear the virus in chronic infection, due to selection pressure exerting on viral

variants, they contribute to the evolution of the HCV envelope sequences to escape (Farci *et al.*, 2000; von Hahn *et al.*, 2007). It has been proposed that HCV stimulates B cells in a B cell receptor-independent manner in chronic infection (Racanelli *et al.*, 2006) and may favor the development of lymphoproliferative and autoimmune diseases (Guidotti & Chisari, 2006).
Although, in vitro studies evident that the neutralization ability of HCV-specific nAbs enhanced by complement activation against pseudotyped viruses (Racanelli *et al.*, 2006), there is absence of direct experimental evidence about the presence of any of these Ab-mediated functions during natural HCV infection. However, immune complexes are believed to play a pathogenetic role in the development of manifestations such as cryoglobulinemia, glomerulonephritis, porphyria cutanea tarda, and necrotizing cutaneous vasculitis during chronic HCV infection (Agnello & De Rosa, 2004; Amarapurkar & Amarapurkar, 2002; Manns & Rambusch, 1999).

3.3.2 Cellular immune response

Cytotoxic T lymphocyte (CTL) responses are essential to control HCV infection. Efficiency of antiviral CTL responses depends on where these cells are primed. Efficient antiviral CTL response is observed when it is primed in lymphoid organs, whereas within the liver, priming is more tend to induce T cell inactivation, tolerance or apoptosis (Guidotti & Chisari, 2006). A strong, multispecific and long-lasting T-cell immune response emerge to be important for control of viral infection (Dustin & Rice, 2007; Zhang *et al.*, 2009). Persistent HCV unsuccessfully control by T effector cells is due to multiple causes, such as: HCV escape mutant generation, immunosuppressive effects exertion, Tregs induction, or effector T cell exhaustion or apoptosis (Bassett *et al.*, 1999; Thimme *et al.*, 2006; Thimme *et al.*, 2001; Larrubia *et al.*, 2011).

3.3.2.1 Adaptive cellular response during acute HCV infection

Vigorous CD4+ and CD8+ T cell responses targeting multiple HCV regions with intrahepatic production of IFN-γ emerged in acute hepatitis C infection (Bowen & Walker, 2005; Lechner *et al.*, 2000b; Thimme *et al.*, 2001). Decreasing viral titer correlates precisely with the appearance of HCV-specific T cells and IFN-γ expression in the liver (Shin *et al.*, 2006). The appearance of HCV-specific T cells can be detectable in the peripheral blood or in the liver compartment several weeks after infection in humans or experimental chimpanzee models (Dustin & Rice, 2007; Rehermann, 2009), respective with primary peak of transaminases and irrespective of clinical outcome (resolution or chronicity). Delayed emerging of antigen-specific responses are also essential for the HCV control (Rehermann, 2009).
The protective function of CD4+ T cells appear to be due to the production of antiviral cytokines, but also their helping nature to antiviral B cells and in maintenance of CD8+ T cell memory. The HCV clearance has been observed and correlated with vigorous proliferation of specific CD4+ T cells (Diepolder *et al.*, 1995; Missale *et al.*, 1996) with concurrent IL-2 and IFN-γ production (Kaplan *et al.*, 2007; Urbani *et al.*, 2006a). The early sustained development of CD4+ T cell response needs to be successful for viral clearance (Urbani *et al.*, 2006a). Whereas, HCV-specific CD4+ T cell responses are not observed in chronic HCV infection. Moreover, the recurrent viremia has been correlated with loss of previous strong CD4+ T cell responses after several months of viral clearance (Gerlach *et al.*, 1999; Nascimbeni *et al.*, 2003). Studies on the relative importance of CD4 help in spontaneous recovery in acute HCV infection demonstrated that fact (Smyk-Pearson *et al.*, 2008). CTL priming in presence of CD4 help is critical factor in protective function (Urbani *et al.*, 2006a).

On the other hand, the magnitude of CD8+ T cells response in acute HCV infection does not correlate with the clinical or viral outcome (Francavilla *et al.*, 2004; Kaplan *et al.*, 2007; Urbani *et al.*, 2006a). Expression of a dysfunctional phenotype with weak proliferation, low IFN-γ production, impaired cytotoxicity and increased levels of the well known exhausted phenotype programmed death-1 receptor (PD-1) are found in HCV infection, irrespective of infection progression (Bowen *et al.*, 2008; Keir *et al.*, 2007; Nakamoto *et al.*, 2008; Sharpe *et al.*, 2007; Trautmann *et al.*, 2006; Urbani *et al.*, 2006b; Larrubia *et al.*, 2011). Antigen-dependent reactivity of HCV-specific CD8+ T cells has been proved by a rapid decay of CD8+ T cell responses during antiviral therapy (Rahman *et al.*, 2004). However, the appearance of self-sustaining memory T cells (CD127+ memory HCV-specific CD8+ T cells and CD4+ T cells) are necessary to control HCV infection (Lechner *et al.*, 2000b; Thimme *et al.*, 2001; Urbani *et al.*, 2006a). In fact, years after HCV control due to anti-HCV treatment it is possible to find HCV traces in association with HCV-specific T cell reactivity. These data suggest that HCV-specific memory T cells are essential to clear HCV infection completely after the initial acute clearing (Veerapu *et al.*, 2011).

3.3.2.2 Adaptive cellular response during chronic HCV infection

Complete resolved HCV patients exhibit broader CTL responses with higher functional avidity and wider cross-recognition ability than patients with persistent HCV infection (Yerly *et al.*, 2008). There are evidences that demonstrate rapid mutation in HCV genome, T cell exhaustion because of expression of inhibitory molecules (Fig.-4), immune regulatory cytokine induction and immune modulatory T reg cell activation, which are main reasons for HCV persistence in chronically infected patients (Hiroishi *et al.*2010; Pavio & Lai, 2003; Seifert *et al.*, 2004; Tester *et al.*, 2005; Larrubia *et al.*, 2011).

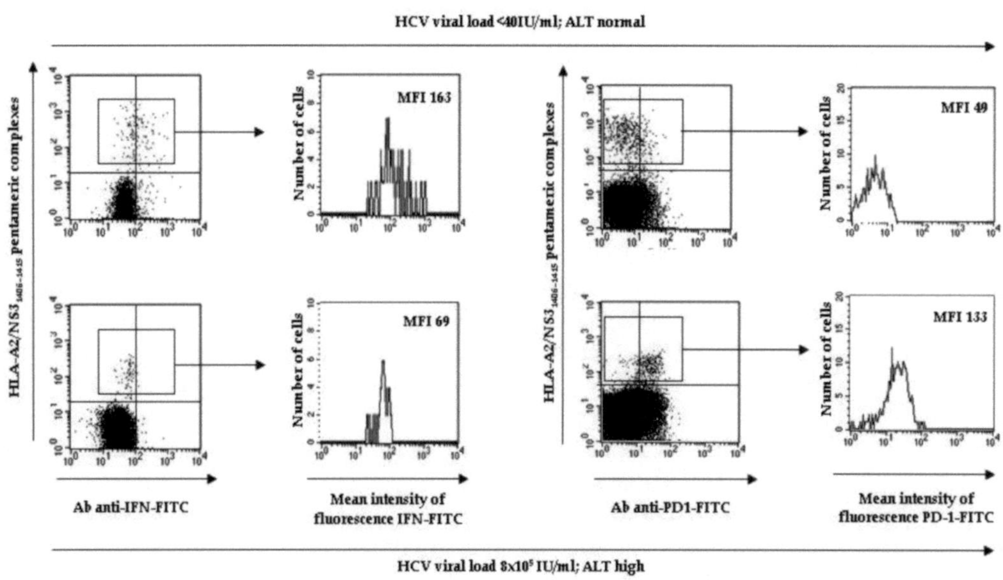

Fig. 4. FACS® dot-plots and histogramas of CD8+ cells from HCV patients with different viral control. CD8+ cells were stained with Abs anti IFN-gamma and anti-PD-1 plus pentemeric HLA-A2/NS3-1406 peptide complexes. A negative correlation between PD-1 expression and IFN-gamma production by HCV-specific T cells according to viral control is shown.

Like Retrovirus, HCV polymerase has high replication rate and lack of proofreading capacity, which permit a rapid virus escape from emerging humoral and cellular immune responses and lead to persistent infection (Chang *et al.*, 1997; Tester *et al.*, 2005). Mutation study in early HCV infection in HLA class I restricted epitopes targeted by CD8+ T cells are associated with persistence (Ray *et al.*, 2005; Timm *et al.*, 2004), which proved indirectly that HLA-restricted CD8+ T cells exert selection pressure. Furthermore, the HLA alleles can influence infection outcome (Neumann-Haefelin *et al.*, 2006).

The secretion of certain immuno-regulatory cytokines is also related with HCV persistence. IL-10 cytokine is found to increase in chronic HCV infection (Piazzolla *et al.*, 2000). In chronic HCV patients, the suppression of IFN-γ production and proliferation of virus-specific CD4+ and CD8+ T cells have been observed in livers with IL-10–producing HCV-specific CD8+ T cells (Accapezzato *et al.*, 2004). IL-10 produced by monocytes or NK cells downregulates effector T cell responses. For instance, monocytes secrete IL-10 in response to HCV core–mediated TLR2 stimulation in vitro (Dolganiuc *et al.*, 2006). IL-10 producing HCV-specific CD8+ T cells inhibits IFN-α production (Duramad *et al.*, 2003), but also promotes apoptosis of pDCs (Dolganiuc *et al.*, 2006), and induces liver infiltration of chronically infected individuals, suggesting that they modulate liver immunopathology to favor HCV persistence (Accapezzato *et al.*, 2004). In addition, intrahepatic HCV-specific IL-10 producing CD8+ T cells prevent liver damage during chronic disease (Abel *et al.*, 2006). Moreover, TGF-b is also involved in antiviral immune suppression and chronic HCV infection evolution (Alatrakchi *et al.*, 2007). To sum up these data, regulatory cytokines such as IL-10 or TGF-beta decrease liver inflammation, after affecting the protective immune response, developing a dual task. First of all, they impair T cell responses to allow viral persistence but also decrease liver damage to extend host survival.

Regulatory T cells (Tregs) are important to control the balance between host damage and viral control produced by specific immune response. In cases of excessive immune response, that could be harmful for the host, these cells can induce immune-tolerance to the viral epitopes. Tregs are derived from natural or induced T cell populations, in which natural CD4+ Tregs are generated during normal T cell development in the thymus, whereas induced Tregs are generated from mature T cells (Bluestone & Abbas, 2003). T cell subset with suppressive function, CD4+ CD25+ FoxP3+ regulatory T (Treg) cells, engages in the control of auto-immunity and immune responses, through various mechanisms including the inhibition of APC maturation and T-cell activation (Shevach, 2009). No difference has been found in the frequency of Treg cells and the extent of suppression irrespective of the outcome of the infection (Manigold *et al.*, 2006). However, higher Tregs frequency has been observed in chronic HCV infected patients than in resolved patients (Boettler *et al.*, 2005; Cabrera *et al.*, 2004; Rushbrook *et al.*, 2005; Sugimoto *et al.*, 2003). Interestingly, depletion of CD25+ cells could enhance responsiveness of the remaining HCV-specific effector cells in vitro (Boettler *et al.*, 2005; Cabrera *et al.*, 2004; Sugimoto *et al.*, 2003), which suggest a fundamental role of Tregs in the establishment of chronic HCV infection. Moreover, Treg cells are induced and proliferate in chronic HCV infection and appeared to alter liver inflammation (Zerbini *et al.*, 2008). Conversely, Programmed Death ligand-1 (PDL-1) mediated inhibition limits the expansion of Tregs by controlling STAT-5 phosphorylation (pSTAT-5) (Franceschini *et al.*, 2009), which can diminish suppressive function of Tregs, lead to viral load control and ultimately ensure long-lasting survival of the host.

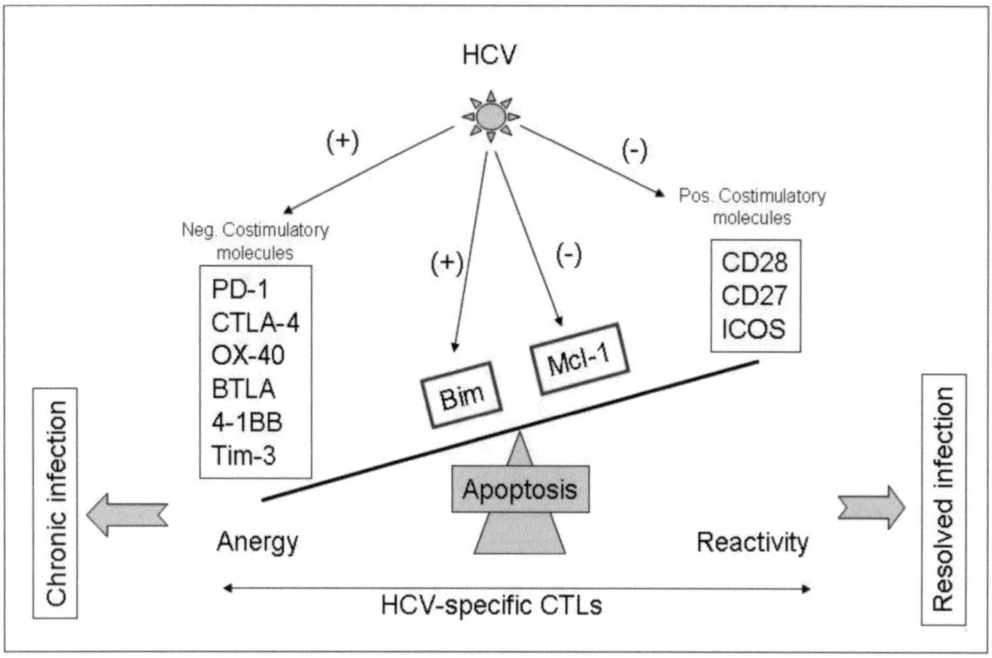

Fig. 5. Scheme showing the balance between co-stimulatory/apoptotic molecules and HCV-specific CTLs reactivity according to infection outcome. Neg.: negative. Pos.: positive. CTLs: cytotoxic T lymphocytes. HCV: hepatitis C virus. (+): possible molecules induced by HCV infection. (-): possible molecules down-regulated by HCV infection.

HCV is able to induce the up-regulation of different negative co-stimulatory molecules in order to provoke an anergic status on HCV-specific T cells. Expression of the inhibitory receptor PD-1 is one of these molecules involved in the generation of a state of exhaustion on HCV-specific CD8+ T cells during chronic HCV infection (Barber *et al.*, 2006; Larrubia *et al.*, 2009b). Importance of expression of PD-1 in HCV-specific T cell failure mechanism has been observed (Golden-Mason *et al.*, 2007; Radziewicz *et al.*, 2007), which can hinder by mutation in T cell epitopes (Rutebemberwa *et al.*, 2008). In addition, blocking of PD-1 signaling resulted in the functional restoration of blood-derived HCV-specific $CD8^+$ T cell responses in chronic infection (Penna *et al.*, 2007; Radziewicz *et al.*, 2007). However, the PD-1 alone is not sufficient in defining exhausted HCV-specific $CD8^+$ T cells during HCV infection. To restore function of HCV-specific T cells isolated from liver biopsies of infected patients, there is need of CTLA4 blockade in addition to PD-1 blockade (Nakamoto *et al.*, 2009). In addition, the co-expression of other inhibitory receptors such as 2B4, CD160, Tim-3 and KLRG1 occurred in about half of HCV-specific CD8+ T cell responses and correlate with low or intermediate level of CD127 expression, impaired proliferative capacity, an intermediate T cell differentiation stage (Bengsch *et al.*, 2010). These data indicates that HCV infection modulates different negative co-stimulatory molecules to favor the development of HCV-specific $CD8^+$ T cell exhaustion. On the other hand, HCV infection is also able to regulate pro-apototic pathways to induce HCV-specific T cell deletion in order to escape from immune response. HCV-specific CTLs from chronic patients targeting the virus express an exhausted phenotype associated to the up-regulation of the pro-apototic molecule Bim. The activity of this molecule is contra-regulated by the anti-apoptotic molecule Mcl-1. Interestingly, the reactivity of these cells is impaired but can be restored by blocking apoptotic pathways (Larrubia *et al.*, 2011).

In summary, HCV is able to impair adaptive immune response at different levels. The effector population in charged of HCV clearing is defective because HCV is able to induce on those cells anergy and apoptosis (Fig.-5). Moreover, HCV is able to escape humoral response and cellular response by escape mutations in immunodominant epitopes. Finally, HCV is also quite efficient in the impairment of the specific T helper response, which is essential to organize the humoral and cellular response. To perform all these immune-escape strategies, HCV takes advantage of the pro-anergenic environment of the infected liver, because HCV-specific T cell priming at this level is not efficient to develop adequate effector cells. As it was commented for HBV infection, HCV immune response restoration could be an interesting therapeutic tool to help in viral clearance in chronic patients.

4. Accepted model of HBV&HCV pathogenesis

As previously commented, specific CTLs play a central role in HBV&HCV immunopathogenesis. These cells are able to kill some infected hepatocytes inducing a minor liver damage, but also they secrete type-I cytokines responsible for non-cytopathic virus clearing. To attract these cells into the liver the infected hepatocytes secrete another kind of cytokines called chemokines. The migration of lymphocytes to the liver is a complex process including adhesion, rolling, triggering, and transendothelial migration. Chemokines and their receptors play an essential role in this multistep pathway (Springer, 1994). During primoinfection, when the adaptive immune system is not able to control infection, the infected hepatocytes continue secreting chemokines to try to attract more defensive cells. In viral chronic hepatitis, the expression of different chemokines in the liver has been described. CXCL-10 is increased in the liver and peripheral blood during viral chronic hepatitis (Larrubia *et al.*, 2007; Shields *et al.*, 1999; Tan *et al.*, 2010; Wang *et al.*, 2008). This molecule is produced by hepatocytes and sinusoidal endothelial cells. Moreover, CXCL9 and CXCL11 are also increased in serum and liver of subjects with chronic viral hepatitis (Bieche *et al.*, 2005). CXCL9 is detected primarily on sinusoidal endothelial cells, while CXCL-11 is produced mainly by hepatocytes (Apolinario *et al.*, 2002). CCL5 intrahepatic expression is also elevated in viral chronic hepatitis and is produced by hepatocytes, sinusoidal endothelial cells and biliary epithelium. Finally, several studies have reported an increased level of CCL3 and CCL4 either in the liver or in serum. These molecules are detected on endothelial cells, on some hepatocytes and biliary epithelial cells (Apolinario *et al.*, 2004). The expression of all these chemokines in the liver can be induced directly by viral proteins. Previous reports have shown a high hepatocyte synthesis of CXCL10, CXCL9 and CCL5, induced by some HCV proteins such as NS5A and core (Apolinario *et al.*, 2005), although a recent in-vitro study suggests that HCV proteins could also decrease CCL5 and CXCL10 genes expression (Sillanpaa *et al.*, 2008). All these chemokines recruit T cells with a Th1/Tc1 phenotype, expressing specific chemokine receptors such as CCR5 and CXCR3. The non-ELR-CXC chemokine attracts CXCR3 expressing T cells while CC chemokine attract CCR5 expressing T cells to the liver. Consequently, in viral chronic hepatitis, an intrahepatic enrichment of CCR5 and CXCR3 expressing T cells, located in hepatic lobule and portal tracts has been shown, while these populations are very infrequent in uninfected subjects (Bertoletti & Maini, 2000; Larrubia *et al.*, 2008) (Fig.- 6).

Persistent HBV&HCV infection is characterized by a non-specific inflammatory infiltrate in the liver, mainly of CD8+ cells (Sprengers *et al.*, 2005), responsible for liver damage. These cells are attracted by the interaction between the intrahepatic secreted chemokines and the chemokine receptors expressed on T cells. Actually, previous reports have shown a correlation between liver inflammation and liver infiltrating CXCR3/CCR5 expressing T cells. The frequency of these cells was positively correlated with portal and lobular inflammation but not with liver fibrosis (Larrubia *et al.*, 2007). These data suggest that CCR5 and CXCR3 could play an important role in chronic liver damage by means of inflammatory T cells recruitment into the liver. Moreover, several previous studies have also shown a correlation between liver inflammation and chemokine levels. Intrahepatic CXCL10 mRNA levels are associated with intralobular inflammation (Harvey *et al.*, 2003). Similarly, CXCL9 and CXCL11 correlate with the grade of liver inflammation (Helbig *et al.*, 2004). Furthermore, CC chemokines are also correlated with the intrahepatic inflammatory activity (Kusano *et al.*, 2000). Clearly, intrahepatic CCL5 positive cells correlate with the inflammatory activity. Bearing in mind all the previous data it is possible to speculate that

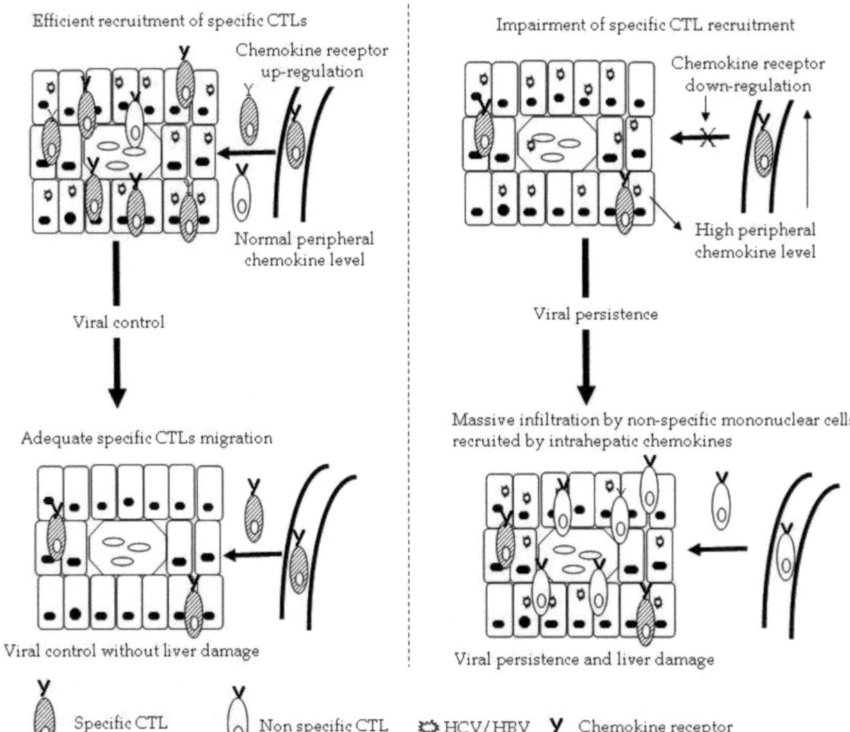

Fig. 6. Scheme showing the role of T cell intrahepatic recruitment according to the degree of liver damage and viral control. In resolved HBV/HCV infection an adequate effector T cell response is attracted to the liver to clear the virus. After that, a memory T cell population is continuously patrolling the liver to keep under control viral traces. Nevertheless, in persistent infection after specific T cells failure to control infection, a non-specific immflamatory infiltrate is sequestered into the liver, responsible of the persistent liver damage.

chemokines are secreted in the infected liver to attract an adaptive immune response able to clear the virus. Unfortunately, when the specific response fails these chemokines also attract non-specific mononuclear and polymorphonuclear cells, which are not able to remove the virus but produce liver inflammation (Kakimi *et al.*, 2001). Therefore, as chemokines are nonspecific chemoattractants, intrahepatic inflammatory infiltrate during chronic infection is mainly non-virus-specific and consequently unable to eliminate the infection, but able to produce cytokines capable of initiating and perpetuating hepatic fibrogenesis (Bertoletti & Maini, 2000; Bertoletti *et al.*, 2010; Friedman, 2003; Larrubia *et al.*, 2008).

5. Mechanisms to restore adaptive immune response in HBV&HCV infection

Bearing in mind that specific T responses are essential to control HCV during natural immune response, several studies have been performed to analyze the role of different therapeutic approaches on T cell response to know whether it is possible to reverse T cell dysfunction in-vivo. Longitudinal analysis of HBV-specific responses during IFN-α treatment did not show a significant increase of these responses during treatment (Sprengers *et al.*, 2007). Nevertheless, it was observed an improvement after treatment in patients with resolved infection (Carotenuto *et al.*, 2009). During HCV infection, the same scenario was observed (Barnes *et al.*, 2002), although some studies have demonstrated a restoration of T cell response in sustained viral responders (Kamal *et al.*, 2002). However, patients presenting a better HCV-specific CD8 cell proliferative potential at baseline, are more likely to present a rapid and sustained viral response. Moreover, after treatment a HCV-specific T-cell response enhancement is observed in sustained viral responders (Pilli *et al.*, 2007). The absence of T cell reactivity improvement during treatment could be due to the direct anti-proliferative effect of IFN-α. Obviously, this effect could counteract the positive consequence of decreasing viral pressure on specific-T cells during treatment. Nevertheless, these data also could suggest that is important to restore a specific T cell response, at least at the end of treatment, to keep under control residual viral traces. In HBV infection, several papers dealing with the role of nucleot(s)ide analogues (NUCs) treatment on anti-HBV immune response have shown that they are able to reconstitute temporally HBV-specific CD4 and CD8 responses (Boni *et al.*, 1998; Cooksley *et al.*, 2008). Moreover, these treatments can decrease the frequency of Tregs during treatment (Stoop *et al.*, 2007) and specifically to decrease the ratio Treg:Th17 (Zhang *et al.*, 2010). These data suggest that the NUCs are controlling the infection not only through an anti-viral effect but also helping to restore specific immune response. In any case, all these effects on specific T cells are partial and limited in time. For that reason other immunoregulatory therapeutic approaches are being considered. Several pre-clinical studies have been performed to try to restore HBV/HCV specific responses in-vitro and in animal models. Modulation of negative co-stimulatory molecules, in addition to blocking immunosupressive cytokines could be promising strategies to restore an effective T cell response. The modulation of negative co-stimulatory molecules, such as PD-1, CTLA-4, Tim-3, has shown in-vitro to increase specific-T cell reactivity. This can be also enhanced using Abs to block the regulatory cytokine IL-10. Experts in immunotherapy have suggested that after restoring a T cell response could be necessary to boost that response using a therapeutic vaccine. Although these results seem to be quite promising, the blockade of negative co-stimulatory pathways in addition to IL-10 could lead to the development of autoimmune diseases, which could prevent the use of this strategy as a therapeutic tool in humans. Therefore, more research is necessary in this field before these strategies are suitable for the treatment of chronic viral infections (Ferrari, 2008; Fisicaro *et al.*, 2010; Larrubia *et al.*, 2011; Nakamoto *et al.*, 2009).

6. Conclusions

HBV & HCV are two hepatotropic non-cytopathic viruses able to develop a chronic liver disease. The innate immune response is defective in both infections, residing the viral control in the efficacy of adaptive immune response. HBV&HCV specific CTL response play a central role in viral control through cytopathic and non-cytopathic mechanisms. Nevertheless, during persistent infection, adaptive response is impaired due to exhaustion and deletion. Several in-vitro strategies have shown to be effective in its restoration but it is necessary more research before these approaches can be applied to clinical practice. Finally, when the virus is not controlled by adaptive response a non-specific inflammatory infiltrate is attracted to the liver which is responsible for the persistent low-grade liver damage, allowing the generation of liver fibrosis during disease progression.

7. Acknowledgments

This book chapter was supported by grants from "Fiscam" (PI-2007/32), (PI-2010/022) and "Fundación de Investigación Médica Mutua Madrileña" (2548/2008), Spain. Benito S and Lokhande MU were supported by research grants from "Fiscam" (MOV-2007_JI/18) and, "Asociación de Hepatología Translacional" (AHT10/01) Spain, respectively.

8. References

Abel, M., Sene, D., Pol, S., Bourliere, M., Poynard, T., Charlotte, F., Cacoub, P. & Caillat-Zucman, S. (2006). Intrahepatic virus-specific IL-10-producing CD8 T cells prevent liver damage during chronic hepatitis C virus infection. *Hepatology* 44, 1607-1616.

Accapezzato, D., Francavilla, V., Paroli, M., Casciaro, M., Chircu, L. V., Cividini, A., Abrignani, S., Mondelli, M. U. & Barnaba, V. (2004). Hepatic expansion of a virus-specific regulatory CD8(+) T cell population in chronic hepatitis C virus infection. *J Clin Invest* 113, 963-972.

Agnello, V., Abel, G., Elfahal, M., Knight, G. B. & Zhang, Q. X. (1999). Hepatitis C virus and other flaviviridae viruses enter cells via low density lipoprotein receptor. *Proc Natl Acad Sci U S A* 96, 12766-12771.

Agnello, V. & De Rosa, F. G. (2004). Extrahepatic disease manifestations of HCV infection: some current issues. *J Hepatol* 40, 341-352.

Ahlenstiel, G., Titerence, R. H., Koh, C., Edlich, B., Feld, J. J., Rotman, Y., Ghany, M. G., Hoofnagle, J. H., Liang, T. J., Heller, T. & Rehermann, B. (2010). Natural killer cells are polarized toward cytotoxicity in chronic hepatitis C in an interferon-alfa-dependent manner. *Gastroenterology* 138, 325-335.

Alatrakchi, N., Graham, C. S., van der Vliet, H. J., Sherman, K. E., Exley, M. A. & Koziel, M. J. (2007). Hepatitis C virus (HCV)-specific CD8+ cells produce transforming growth factor beta that can suppress HCV-specific T-cell responses. *J Virol* 81, 5882-5892.

Albert, M. L., Decalf, J. & Pol, S. (2008). Plasmacytoid dendritic cells move down on the list of suspects: in search of the immune pathogenesis of chronic hepatitis C. *J Hepatol* 49, 1069-1078.

Alexopoulou, L., Holt, A. C., Medzhitov, R. & Flavell, R. A. (2001). Recognition of double-stranded RNA and activation of NF-kappaB by Toll-like receptor 3. *Nature* 413, 732-738.

Alter, H. J., Purcell, R. H., Holland, P. V. & Popper, H. (1978). Transmissible agent in non-A, non-B hepatitis. *Lancet* 1, 459-463.

Amarapurkar, D. N. & Amarapurkar, A. D. (2002). Extrahepatic manifestations of viral hepatitis. *Ann Hepatol* 1, 192-195.

Anthony, D. D., Yonkers, N. L., Post, A. B., Asaad, R., Heinzel, F. P., Lederman, M. M., Lehmann, P. V. & Valdez, H. (2004). Selective impairments in dendritic cell-associated function distinguish hepatitis C virus and HIV infection. *J Immunol* 172, 4907-4916.

Apolinario, A., Diago, M., Lo Iacono, O., Lorente, R., Perez, C., Majano, P. L., Clemente, G. & Garcia-Monzon, C. (2004). Increased circulating and intrahepatic T-cell-specific chemokines in chronic hepatitis C: relationship with the type of virological response to peginterferon plus ribavirin combination therapy. *Aliment Pharmacol Ther* 19, 551-562.

Apolinario, A., Majano, P. L., Alvarez-Perez, E., Saez, A., Lozano, C., Vargas, J. & Garcia-Monzon, C. (2002). Increased expression of T cell chemokines and their receptors in chronic hepatitis C: relationship with the histological activity of liver disease. *Am J Gastroenterol* 97, 2861-2870.

Apolinario, A., Majano, P. L., Lorente, R., Nunez, O., Clemente, G. & Garcia-Monzon, C. (2005). Gene expression profile of T-cell-specific chemokines in human hepatocyte-derived cells: evidence for a synergistic inducer effect of cytokines and hepatitis C virus proteins. *J Viral Hepat* 12, 27-37.

Appay, V., van Lier, R. A., Sallusto, F. & Roederer, M. (2008). Phenotype and function of human T lymphocyte subsets: consensus and issues. *Cytometry A* 73, 975-983.

Barber, D. L., Wherry, E. J., Masopust, D., Zhu, B., Allison, J. P., Sharpe, A. H., Freeman, G. J. & Ahmed, R. (2006). Restoring function in exhausted CD8 T cells during chronic viral infection. *Nature* 439, 682-687.

Barnes, E., Harcourt, G., Brown, D., Lucas, M., Phillips, R., Dusheiko, G. & Klenerman, P. (2002). The dynamics of T-lymphocyte responses during combination therapy for chronic hepatitis C virus infection. *Hepatology* 36, 743-754.

Barton, G. M. (2007). Viral recognition by Toll-like receptors. *Semin Immunol* 19, 33-40.

Bartosch, B., Dubuisson, J. & Cosset, F. L. (2003a). Infectious hepatitis C virus pseudo-particles containing functional E1-E2 envelope protein complexes. *J Exp Med* 197, 633-642.

Bartosch, B., Vitelli, A., Granier, C., Goujon, C., Dubuisson, J., Pascale, S., Scarselli, E., Cortese, R., Nicosia, A. & Cosset, F. L. (2003b). Cell entry of hepatitis C virus requires a set of co-receptors that include the CD81 tetraspanin and the SR-B1 scavenger receptor. *J Biol Chem* 278, 41624-41630.

Bassett, S. E., Thomas, D. L., Brasky, K. M. & Lanford, R. E. (1999). Viral persistence, antibody to E1 and E2, and hypervariable region 1 sequence stability in hepatitis C virus-inoculated chimpanzees. *J Virol* 73, 1118-1126.

Bauer, S., Kirschning, C. J., Hacker, H., Redecke, V., Hausmann, S., Akira, S., Wagner, H. & Lipford, G. B. (2001). Human TLR9 confers responsiveness to bacterial DNA via species-specific CpG motif recognition. *Proc Natl Acad Sci U S A* 98, 9237-9242.

Baumert, T. F., Ito, S., Wong, D. T. & Liang, T. J. (1998). Hepatitis C virus structural proteins assemble into viruslike particles in insect cells. *J Virol* 72, 3827-3836.

Benedicto, I., Molina-Jimenez, F., Bartosch, B., Cosset, F. L., Lavillette, D., Prieto, J., Moreno-Otero, R., Valenzuela-Fernandez, A., Aldabe, R., Lopez-Cabrera, M. & Majano, P. L. (2009). The tight junction-associated protein occludin is required for a postbinding step in hepatitis C virus entry and infection. *J Virol* 83, 8012-8020.

Bengsch, B., Seigel, B., Ruhl, M., Timm, J., Kuntz, M., Blum, H. E., Pircher, H. & Thimme, R. (2010). Coexpression of PD-1, 2B4, CD160 and KLRG1 on exhausted HCV-specific CD8+ T cells is linked to antigen recognition and T cell differentiation. *PLoS Pathog* 6, e1000947.

Bertoletti, A. & Maini, M. K. (2000). Protection or damage: a dual role for the virus-specific cytotoxic T lymphocyte response in hepatitis B and C infection?. *Curr Opin Microbiol* 3, 387-392.

Bertoletti, A., Maini, M. K. & Ferrari, C. (2010). The host-pathogen interaction during HBV infection: immunological controversies. *Antivir Ther* 15 Suppl 3, 15-24.

Bieche, I., Asselah, T., Laurendeau, I., Vidaud, D., Degot, C., Paradis, V., Bedossa, P., Valla, D. C., Marcellin, P. & Vidaud, M. (2005). Molecular profiling of early stage liver fibrosis in patients with chronic hepatitis C virus infection. *Virology* 332, 130-144.

Biron, C. A., Nguyen, K. B., Pien, G. C., Cousens, L. P. & Salazar-Mather, T. P. (1999). Natural killer cells in antiviral defense: function and regulation by innate cytokines. *Annu Rev Immunol* 17, 189-220.

Blanchard, E., Belouzard, S., Goueslain, L., Wakita, T., Dubuisson, J., Wychowski, C. & Rouille, Y. (2006). Hepatitis C virus entry depends on clathrin-mediated endocytosis. *J Virol* 80, 6964-6972.

Blight, K. J., Kolykhalov, A. A. & Rice, C. M. (2000). Efficient initiation of HCV RNA replication in cell culture. *Science* 290, 1972-1974.

Blight, K. J., McKeating, J. A., Marcotrigiano, J. & Rice, C. M. (2003). Efficient replication of hepatitis C virus genotype 1a RNAs in cell culture. *J Virol* 77, 3181-3190.

Blight, K. J., McKeating, J. A. & Rice, C. M. (2002). Highly permissive cell lines for subgenomic and genomic hepatitis C virus RNA replication. *J Virol* 76, 13001-13014.

Bluestone, J. A. & Abbas, A. K. (2003). Natural versus adaptive regulatory T cells. *Nat Rev Immunol* 3, 253-257.

Bode, J. G., Ludwig, S., Ehrhardt, C., Albrecht, U., Erhardt, A., Schaper, F., Heinrich, P. C. & Haussinger, D. (2003). IFN-alpha antagonistic activity of HCV core protein involves induction of suppressor of cytokine signaling-3. *FASEB J* 17, 488-490.

Boettler, T., Spangenberg, H. C., Neumann-Haefelin, C., Panther, E., Urbani, S., Ferrari, C., Blum, H. E., von Weizsacker, F. & Thimme, R. (2005). T cells with a CD4+CD25+ regulatory phenotype suppress in vitro proliferation of virus-specific CD8+ T cells during chronic hepatitis C virus infection. *J Virol* 79, 7860-7867.

Boni, C., Bertoletti, A., Penna, A., Cavalli, A., Pilli, M., Urbani, S., Scognamiglio, P., Boehme, R., Panebianco, R., Fiaccadori, F. & Ferrari, C. (1998). Lamivudine treatment can restore T cell responsiveness in chronic hepatitis B. *J Clin Invest* 102, 968-975.

Boni, C., Fisicaro, P., Valdatta, C., Amadei, B., Di Vincenzo, P., Giuberti, T., Laccabue, D., Zerbini, A., Cavalli, A., Missale, G., Bertoletti, A. & Ferrari, C. (2007). Characterization of hepatitis B virus (HBV)-specific T-cell dysfunction in chronic HBV infection. *J Virol* 81, 4215-4225.

Bowen, D. G., Shoukry, N. H., Grakoui, A., Fuller, M. J., Cawthon, A. G., Dong, C., Hasselschwert, D. L., Brasky, K. M., Freeman, G. J., Seth, N. P., Wucherpfennig, K. W., Houghton, M. & Walker, C. M. (2008). Variable patterns of programmed death-1 expression on fully functional memory T cells after spontaneous resolution of hepatitis C virus infection. *J Virol* 82, 5109-5114.

Bowen, D. G. & Walker, C. M. (2005). Adaptive immune responses in acute and chronic hepatitis C virus infection. *Nature* 436, 946-952.

Bukh, J. (2004). A critical role for the chimpanzee model in the study of hepatitis C. *Hepatology* 39, 1469-1475.

Cabrera, R., Tu, Z., Xu, Y., Firpi, R. J., Rosen, H. R., Liu, C. & Nelson, D. R. (2004). An immunomodulatory role for CD4(+)CD25(+) regulatory T lymphocytes in hepatitis C virus infection. *Hepatology* 40, 1062-1071.

Carotenuto, P., Artsen, A., Niesters, H. G., Osterhaus, A. D. & Pontesilli, O. (2009). In vitro use of autologous dendritic cells improves detection of T cell responses to hepatitis B virus (HBV) antigens. *J Med Virol* 81, 332-339.

Cooksley, H., Chokshi, S., Maayan, Y., Wedemeyer, H., Andreone, P., Gilson, R., Warnes, T., Paganin, S., Zoulim, F., Frederick, D., Neumann, A. U., Brosgart, C. L. & Naoumov, N. V. (2008). Hepatitis B virus e antigen loss during adefovir dipivoxil therapy is associated with enhanced virus-specific CD4+ T-cell reactivity. *Antimicrob Agents Chemother* 52, 312-320.

Chang, K. M., Rehermann, B., McHutchison, J. G., Pasquinelli, C., Southwood, S., Sette, A. & Chisari, F. V. (1997). Immunological significance of cytotoxic T lymphocyte epitope variants in patients chronically infected by the hepatitis C virus. *J Clin Invest* 100, 2376-2385.

Chen, Z., Cheng, Y., Xu, Y., Liao, J., Zhang, X., Hu, Y., Zhang, Q., Wang, J., Zhang, Z., Shen, F. & Yuan, Z. (2008). Expression profiles and function of Toll-like receptors 2 and 4 in peripheral blood mononuclear cells of chronic hepatitis B patients. *Clin Immunol* 128, 400-408.

Choudhuri, K., Kearney, A., Bakker, T. R. & van der Merwe, P. A. (2005). Immunology: how do T cells recognize antigen? *Curr Biol* 15, R382-385.

Das, A., Hoare, M., Davies, N., Lopes, A. R., Dunn, C., Kennedy, P. T., Alexander, G., Finney, H., Lawson, A., Plunkett, F. J., Bertoletti, A., Akbar, A. N. & Maini, M. K. (2008). Functional skewing of the global CD8 T cell population in chronic hepatitis B virus infection. *J Exp Med* 205, 2111-2124.

Decalf, J., Fernandes, S., Longman, R., Ahloulay, M., Audat, F., Lefrerre, F., Rice, C. M., Pol, S. & Albert, M. L. (2007). Plasmacytoid dendritic cells initiate a complex chemokine and cytokine network and are a viable drug target in chronic HCV patients. *J Exp Med* 204, 2423-2437.

Diepolder, H. M., Zachoval, R., Hoffmann, R. M., Wierenga, E. A., Santantonio, T., Jung, M. C., Eichenlaub, D. & Pape, G. R. (1995). Possible mechanism involving T-lymphocyte response to non-structural protein 3 in viral clearance in acute hepatitis C virus infection. *Lancet* 346, 1006-1007.

Dolganiuc, A., Chang, S., Kodys, K., Mandrekar, P., Bakis, G., Cormier, M. & Szabo, G. (2006). Hepatitis C virus (HCV) core protein-induced, monocyte-mediated mechanisms of reduced IFN-alpha and plasmacytoid dendritic cell loss in chronic HCV infection. *J Immunol* 177, 6758-6768.

Dunn, C., Brunetto, M., Reynolds, G., Christophides, T., Kennedy, P. T., Lampertico, P., Das, A., Lopes, A. R., Borrow, P., Williams, K., Humphreys, E., Afford, S., Adams, D. H., Bertoletti, A. & Maini, M. K. (2007). Cytokines induced during chronic hepatitis B virus infection promote a pathway for NK cell-mediated liver damage. *J Exp Med* 204, 667-680.

Dunn, C., Peppa, D., Khanna, P., Nebbia, G., Jones, M., Brendish, N., Lascar, R. M., Brown, D., Gilson, R. J., Tedder, R. J., Dusheiko, G. M., Jacobs, M., Klenerman, P. & Maini, M. K. (2009). Temporal analysis of early immune responses in patients with acute hepatitis B virus infection. *Gastroenterology* 137, 1289-1300.

Duramad, O., Fearon, K. L., Chan, J. H., Kanzler, H., Marshall, J. D., Coffman, R. L. & Barrat, F. J. (2003). IL-10 regulates plasmacytoid dendritic cell response to CpG-containing immunostimulatory sequences. *Blood* 102, 4487-4492.

Dustin, L. B. & Rice, C. M. (2007). Flying under the radar: the immunobiology of hepatitis C. *Annu Rev Immunol* 25, 71-99.

Evans, M. J., von Hahn, T., Tscherne, D. M., Syder, A. J., Panis, M., Wolk, B., Hatziioannou, T., McKeating, J. A., Bieniasz, P. D. & Rice, C. M. (2007). Claudin-1 is a hepatitis C virus co-receptor required for a late step in entry. *Nature* 446, 801-805.

Farci, P., Shimoda, A., Coiana, A., Diaz, G., Peddis, G., Melpolder, J. C., Strazzera, A., Chien, D. Y., Munoz, S. J., Balestrieri, A., Purcell, R. H. & Alter, H. J. (2000). The outcome of acute hepatitis C predicted by the evolution of the viral quasispecies. *Science* 288, 339-344.

Ferrari, C. (2008). Therapeutic vaccination for hepatitis C: can protective T-cell responses be restored after prolonged antigen exposure?. *Gastroenterology* 134, 1601-1604.

Ferrari, C., Missale, G., Boni, C. & Urbani, S. (2003). Immunopathogenesis of hepatitis B. *J Hepatol* 39 Suppl 1, S36-42.

Fisicaro, P., Valdatta, C., Boni, C., Massari, M., Mori, C., Zerbini, A., Orlandini, A., Sacchelli, L., Missale, G. & Ferrari, C. (2009). Early kinetics of innate and adaptive immune responses during hepatitis B virus infection. *Gut* 58, 974-982.

Fisicaro, P., Valdatta, C., Massari, M., Loggi, E., Biasini, E., Sacchelli, L., Cavallo, M. C., Silini, E. M., Andreone, P., Missale, G. & Ferrari, C. (2010). Antiviral intrahepatic T-cell responses can be restored by blocking programmed death-1 pathway in chronic hepatitis B. *Gastroenterology* 138, 682-693, 693 e681-684.

Fitzgerald-Bocarsly, P., Dai, J. & Singh, S. (2008). Plasmacytoid dendritic cells and type I IFN: 50 years of convergent history. *Cytokine Growth Factor Rev* 19, 3-19.

Foy, E., Li, K., Wang, C., Sumpter, R., Jr., Ikeda, M., Lemon, S. M. & Gale, M., Jr. (2003). Regulation of interferon regulatory factor-3 by the hepatitis C virus serine protease. *Science* 300, 1145-1148.

Francavilla, V., Accapezzato, D., De Salvo, M., Rawson, P., Cosimi, O., Lipp, M., Cerino, A., Cividini, A., Mondelli, M. U. & Barnaba, V. (2004). Subversion of effector CD8+ T cell differentiation in acute hepatitis C virus infection: exploring the immunological mechanisms. *Eur J Immunol* 34, 427-437.

Franceschini, D., Paroli, M., Francavilla, V., Videtta, M., Morrone, S., Labbadia, G., Cerino, A., Mondelli, M. U. & Barnaba, V. (2009). PD-L1 negatively regulates CD4+CD25+Foxp3+ Tregs by limiting STAT-5 phosphorylation in patients chronically infected with HCV. *J Clin Invest* 119, 551-564.

Frelin, L., Wahlstrom, T., Tucker, A. E., Jones, J., Hughes, J., Lee, B. O., Billaud, J. N., Peters, C., Whitacre, D., Peterson, D. & Milich, D. R. (2009). A mechanism to explain the selection of the hepatitis e antigen-negative mutant during chronic hepatitis B virus infection. *J Virol* 83, 1379-1392.

Fried, M. W., Shiffman, M. L., Reddy, K. R., Smith, C., Marinos, G., Goncales, F. L., Jr., Haussinger, D., Diago, M., Carosi, G., Dhumeaux, D., Craxi, A., Lin, A., Hoffman, J. & Yu, J. (2002). Peginterferon alfa-2a plus ribavirin for chronic hepatitis C virus infection. *N Engl J Med* 347, 975-982.

Friedman, S. L. (2003). Liver fibrosis -- from bench to bedside. *J Hepatol* 38 Suppl 1, S38-53.

Furuichi, Y., Tokuyama, H., Ueha, S., Kurachi, M., Moriyasu, F. & Kakimi, K. (2005). Depletion of CD25+CD4+T cells (Tregs) enhances the HBV-specific CD8+ T cell response primed by DNA immunization. *World J Gastroenterol* 11, 3772-3777.

Gal-Tanamy, M., Keck, Z. Y., Yi, M., McKeating, J. A., Patel, A. H., Foung, S. K. & Lemon, S. M. (2008). In vitro selection of a neutralization-resistant hepatitis C virus escape mutant. *Proc Natl Acad Sci U S A* 105, 19450-19455.

Gale, M., Jr. & Foy, E. M. (2005). Evasion of intracellular host defence by hepatitis C virus. *Nature* 436, 939-945.

Garry, R. F. & Dash, S. (2003). Proteomics computational analyses suggest that hepatitis C virus E1 and pestivirus E2 envelope glycoproteins are truncated class II fusion proteins. *Virology* 307, 255-265.

Gealy, C., Denson, M., Humphreys, C., McSharry, B., Wilkinson, G. & Caswell, R. (2005). Posttranscriptional suppression of interleukin-6 production by human cytomegalovirus. *J Virol* 79, 472-485.

Gerlach, J. T., Diepolder, H. M., Jung, M. C., Gruener, N. H., Schraut, W. W., Zachoval, R., Hoffmann, R., Schirren, C. A., Santantonio, T. & Pape, G. R. (1999). Recurrence of hepatitis C virus after loss of virus-specific CD4(+) T-cell response in acute hepatitis C. *Gastroenterology* 117, 933-941.

Golden-Mason, L., Madrigal-Estebas, L., McGrath, E., Conroy, M. J., Ryan, E. J., Hegarty, J. E., O'Farrelly, C. & Doherty, D. G. (2008). Altered natural killer cell subset distributions in resolved and persistent hepatitis C virus infection following single source exposure. *Gut* 57, 1121-1128.

Golden-Mason, L., Palmer, B., Klarquist, J., Mengshol, J. A., Castelblanco, N. & Rosen, H. R. (2007). Upregulation of PD-1 expression on circulating and intrahepatic hepatitis C virus-specific CD8+ T cells associated with reversible immune dysfunction. *J Virol* 81, 9249-9258.

Golden-Mason, L. & Rosen, H. R. (2006). Natural killer cells: primary target for hepatitis C virus immune evasion strategies? *Liver Transpl* 12, 363-372.

Grove, J., Huby, T., Stamataki, Z., Vanwolleghem, T., Meuleman, P., Farquhar, M., Schwarz, A., Moreau, M., Owen, J. S., Leroux-Roels, G., Balfe, P. & McKeating, J. A. (2007). Scavenger receptor BI and BII expression levels modulate hepatitis C virus infectivity. *J Virol* 81, 3162-3169.

Grove, J., Nielsen, S., Zhong, J., Bassendine, M. F., Drummer, H. E., Balfe, P. & McKeating, J. A. (2008). Identification of a residue in hepatitis C virus E2 glycoprotein that determines scavenger receptor BI and CD81 receptor dependency and sensitivity to neutralizing antibodies. *J Virol* 82, 12020-12029.

Guidotti, L. G. & Chisari, F. V. (2001). Noncytolytic control of viral infections by the innate and adaptive immune response. *Annu Rev Immunol* 19, 65-91.

Guidotti, L. G. & Chisari, F. V. (2006). Immunobiology and pathogenesis of viral hepatitis. *Annu Rev Pathol* 1, 23-61.

Guidotti, L. G., Rochford, R., Chung, J., Shapiro, M., Purcell, R. & Chisari, F. V. (1999). Viral clearance without destruction of infected cells during acute HBV infection. *Science* 284, 825-829.

Guy, C. S., Mulrooney-Cousins, P. M., Churchill, N. D. & Michalak, T. I. (2008). Intrahepatic expression of genes affiliated with innate and adaptive immune responses immediately after invasion and during acute infection with woodchuck hepadnavirus. *J Virol* 82, 8579-8591.

Haberstroh, A., Schnober, E. K., Zeisel, M. B., Carolla, P., Barth, H., Blum, H. E., Cosset, F. L., Koutsoudakis, G., Bartenschlager, R., Union, A., Depla, E., Owsianka, A., Patel, A. H., Schuster, C., Stoll-Keller, F., Doffoel, M., Dreux, M. & Baumert, T. F. (2008). Neutralizing host responses in hepatitis C virus infection target viral entry at postbinding steps and membrane fusion. *Gastroenterology* 135, 1719-1728 e1711.

Haid, S., Pietschmann, T. & Pecheur, E. I. (2009). Low pH-dependent hepatitis C virus membrane fusion depends on E2 integrity, target lipid composition, and density of virus particles. *J Biol Chem* 284, 17657-17667.

Harvey, C. E., Post, J. J., Palladinetti, P., Freeman, A. J., Ffrench, R. A., Kumar, R. K., Marinos, G. & Lloyd, A. R. (2003). Expression of the chemokine IP-10 (CXCL10) by hepatocytes in chronic hepatitis C virus infection correlates with histological severity and lobular inflammation. *J Leukoc Biol* 74, 360-369.

Heim, M. H., Moradpour, D. & Blum, H. E. (1999). Expression of hepatitis C virus proteins inhibits signal transduction through the Jak-STAT pathway. *J Virol* 73, 8469-8475.

Helbig, K. J., Ruszkiewicz, A., Semendric, L., Harley, H. A., McColl, S. R. & Beard, M. R. (2004). Expression of the CXCR3 ligand I-TAC by hepatocytes in chronic hepatitis C and its correlation with hepatic inflammation. *Hepatology* 39, 1220-1229.

Hiroishi, K., Eguchi, J., Ishii, S., Hiraide, A., Sakaki, M., Doi, H., Omori, R. & Imawari, M. (2010). Immune response of cytotoxic T lymphocytes and possibility of vaccine development for hepatitis C virus infection. *J Biomed Biotechnol* 2010, 263810.

Honda, K., Yanai, H., Mizutani, T., Negishi, H., Shimada, N., Suzuki, N., Ohba, Y., Takaoka, A., Yeh, W. C. & Taniguchi, T. (2004). Role of a transductional-transcriptional processor complex involving MyD88 and IRF-7 in Toll-like receptor signaling. *Proc Natl Acad Sci U S A* 101, 15416-15421.

Hosel, M., Quasdorff, M., Wiegmann, K., Webb, D., Zedler, U., Broxtermann, M., Tedjokusumo, R., Esser, K., Arzberger, S., Kirschning, C. J., Langenkamp, A., Falk, C., Buning, H., Rose-John, S. & Protzer, U. (2009). Not interferon, but interleukin-6 controls early gene expression in hepatitis B virus infection. *Hepatology* 50, 1773-1782.

Hoshino, K., Sugiyama, T., Matsumoto, M., Tanaka, T., Saito, M., Hemmi, H., Ohara, O., Akira, S. & Kaisho, T. (2006). IkappaB kinase-alpha is critical for interferon-alpha production induced by Toll-like receptors 7 and 9. *Nature* 440, 949-953.

Hsu, M., Zhang, J., Flint, M., Logvinoff, C., Cheng-Mayer, C., Rice, C. M. & McKeating, J. A. (2003). Hepatitis C virus glycoproteins mediate pH-dependent cell entry of pseudotyped retroviral particles. *Proc Natl Acad Sci U S A* 100, 7271-7276.

Ikeda, M., Yi, M., Li, K. & Lemon, S. M. (2002). Selectable subgenomic and genome-length dicistronic RNAs derived from an infectious molecular clone of the HCV-N strain of hepatitis C virus replicate efficiently in cultured Huh7 cells. *J Virol* 76, 2997-3006.

Izaguirre, A., Barnes, B. J., Amrute, S., Yeow, W. S., Megjugorac, N., Dai, J., Feng, D., Chung, E., Pitha, P. M. & Fitzgerald-Bocarsly, P. (2003). Comparative analysis of IRF and IFN-alpha expression in human plasmacytoid and monocyte-derived dendritic cells. *J Leukoc Biol* 74, 1125-1138.

Kakimi, K., Guidotti, L. G., Koezuka, Y. & Chisari, F. V. (2000). Natural killer T cell activation inhibits hepatitis B virus replication in vivo. *J Exp Med* 192, 921-930.

Kakimi, K., Lane, T. E., Wieland, S., Asensio, V. C., Campbell, I. L., Chisari, F. V. & Guidotti, L. G. (2001). Blocking chemokine responsive to gamma-2/interferon (IFN)-gamma inducible protein and monokine induced by IFN-gamma activity in vivo reduces the pathogenetic but not the antiviral potential of hepatitis B virus-specific cytotoxic T lymphocytes. *J Exp Med* 194, 1755-1766.

Kamal, S. M., Fehr, J., Roesler, B., Peters, T. & Rasenack, J. W. (2002). Peginterferon alone or with ribavirin enhances HCV-specific CD4 T-helper 1 responses in patients with chronic hepatitis C. *Gastroenterology* 123, 1070-1083.

Kann, M., Schmitz, A. & Rabe, B. (2007). Intracellular transport of hepatitis B virus. *World J Gastroenterol* 13, 39-47.

Kanto, T., Hayashi, N., Takehara, T., Tatsumi, T., Kuzushita, N., Ito, A., Sasaki, Y., Kasahara, A. & Hori, M. (1999). Impaired allostimulatory capacity of peripheral blood dendritic cells recovered from hepatitis C virus-infected individuals. *J Immunol* 162, 5584-5591.

Kapadia, S. B., Barth, H., Baumert, T., McKeating, J. A. & Chisari, F. V. (2007). Initiation of hepatitis C virus infection is dependent on cholesterol and cooperativity between CD81 and scavenger receptor B type I. *J Virol* 81, 374-383.

Kaplan, D. E., Sugimoto, K., Newton, K., Valiga, M. E., Ikeda, F., Aytaman, A., Nunes, F. A., Lucey, M. R., Vance, B. A., Vonderheide, R. H., Reddy, K. R., McKeating, J. A. & Chang, K. M. (2007). Discordant role of CD4 T-cell response relative to neutralizing antibody and CD8 T-cell responses in acute hepatitis C. *Gastroenterology* 132, 654-666.

Kawaguchi, T., Yoshida, T., Harada, M., Hisamoto, T., Nagao, Y., Ide, T., Taniguchi, E., Kumemura, H., Hanada, S., Maeyama, M., Baba, S., Koga, H., Kumashiro, R., Ueno, T., Ogata, H., Yoshimura, A. & Sata, M. (2004). Hepatitis C virus down-regulates insulin receptor substrates 1 and 2 through up-regulation of suppressor of cytokine signaling 3. *Am J Pathol* 165, 1499-1508.

Kawai, T. & Akira, S. (2008). Toll-like receptor and RIG-I-like receptor signaling. *Ann N Y Acad Sci* 1143, 1-20.

Keck, Z. Y., Li, S. H., Xia, J., von Hahn, T., Balfe, P., McKeating, J. A., Witteveldt, J., Patel, A. H., Alter, H., Rice, C. M. & Foung, S. K. (2009). Mutations in hepatitis C virus E2 located outside the CD81 binding sites lead to escape from broadly neutralizing antibodies but compromise virus infectivity. *J Virol* 83, 6149-6160.

Keir, M. E., Francisco, L. M. & Sharpe, A. H. (2007). PD-1 and its ligands in T-cell immunity. *Curr Opin Immunol* 19, 309-314.

Khakoo, S. I., Thio, C. L., Martin, M. P., Brooks, C. R., Gao, X., Astemborski, J., Cheng, J., Goedert, J. J., Vlahov, D., Hilgartner, M., Cox, S., Little, A. M., Alexander, G. J.,

Cramp, M. E., O'Brien, S. J., Rosenberg, W. M., Thomas, D. L. & Carrington, M. (2004). HLA and NK cell inhibitory receptor genes in resolving hepatitis C virus infection. *Science* 305, 872-874.

Kim, K. I., Giannakopoulos, N. V., Virgin, H. W. & Zhang, D. E. (2004). Interferon-inducible ubiquitin E2, Ubc8, is a conjugating enzyme for protein ISGylation. *Mol Cell Biol* 24, 9592-9600.

Knapp, S., Warshow, U., Hegazy, D., Brackenbury, L., Guha, I. N., Fowell, A., Little, A. M., Alexander, G. J., Rosenberg, W. M., Cramp, M. E. & Khakoo, S. I. (2010). Consistent beneficial effects of killer cell immunoglobulin-like receptor 2DL3 and group 1 human leukocyte antigen-C following exposure to hepatitis C virus. *Hepatology* 51, 1168-1175.

Koutsoudakis, G., Kaul, A., Steinmann, E., Kallis, S., Lohmann, V., Pietschmann, T. & Bartenschlager, R. (2006). Characterization of the early steps of hepatitis C virus infection by using luciferase reporter viruses. *J Virol* 80, 5308-5320.

Koyama, A. H., Irie, H., Fukumori, T., Hata, S., Iida, S., Akari, H. & Adachi, A. (1998). Role of virus-induced apoptosis in a host defense mechanism against virus infection. *J Med Invest* 45, 37-45.

Kusano, F., Tanaka, Y., Marumo, F. & Sato, C. (2000). Expression of C-C chemokines is associated with portal and periportal inflammation in the liver of patients with chronic hepatitis C. *Lab Invest* 80, 415-422.

Lang, T., Lo, C., Skinner, N., Locarnini, S., Visvanathan, K. & Mansell, A. (2011) The Hepatitis B e antigen (HBeAg) targets and suppresses activation of the Toll-like receptor signaling pathway. *J Hepatol.* In press.

Lanzavecchia, A. & Sallusto, F. (2001). Regulation of T cell immunity by dendritic cells. *Cell* 106, 263-266.

Larrea, E., Riezu-Boj, J. I., Gil-Guerrero, L., Casares, N., Aldabe, R., Sarobe, P., Civeira, M. P., Heeney, J. L., Rollier, C., Verstrepen, B., Wakita, T., Borras-Cuesta, F., Lasarte, J. J. & Prieto, J. (2007). Upregulation of indoleamine 2,3-dioxygenase in hepatitis C virus infection. *J Virol* 81, 3662-3666.

Larrubia, J. R. (2011). Occult hepatitis B virus infection: a complex entity with relevant clinical implications. *World J Gastroenterol* 17, 1529-1530.

Larrubia, J. R., Benito-Martinez, S., Calvino, M., Sanz-de-Villalobos, E. & Parra-Cid, T. (2008). Role of chemokines and their receptors in viral persistence and liver damage during chronic hepatitis C virus infection. *World J Gastroenterol* 14, 7149-7159.

Larrubia, J. R., Benito-Martinez, S., Miquel-Plaza, J., Sanz-de-Villalobos, E., Gonzalez-Mateos, F. & Parra, T. (2009a). Cytokines - their pathogenic and therapeutic role in chronic viral hepatitis. *Rev Esp Enferm Dig* 101, 343-351.

Larrubia, J. R., Benito-Martinez, S., Miquel, J., Calvino, M., Sanz-de-Villalobos, E., Gonzalez-Praetorius, A., Albertos, S., Garcia-Garzon, S., Lokhande, M. & Parra-Cid, T. (2011). Bim-mediated apoptosis and PD-1/PD-L1 pathway impair reactivity of PD1(+)/CD127(-) HCV-specific CD8(+) cells targeting the virus in chronic hepatitis C virus infection. *Cell Immunol* 269, 104-114.

Larrubia, J. R., Benito-Martinez, S., Miquel, J., Calvino, M., Sanz-de-Villalobos, E. & Parra-Cid, T. (2009b). Costimulatory molecule programmed death-1 in the cytotoxic response during chronic hepatitis C. *World J Gastroenterol.* 15, 5129-5140.

Larrubia, J. R., Calvino, M., Benito, S., Sanz-de-Villalobos, E., Perna, C., Perez-Hornedo, J., Gonzalez-Mateos, F., Garcia-Garzon, S., Bienvenido, A. & Parra, T. (2007). The role of CCR5/CXCR3 expressing CD8+ cells in liver damage and viral control during persistent hepatitis C virus infection. *J Hepatol* 47, 632-641.

Lavanchy, D. (2009). The global burden of hepatitis C. *Liver Int* 29 Suppl 1, 74-81.

Lavillette, D., Bartosch, B., Nourrisson, D., Verney, G., Cosset, F. L., Penin, F. & Pecheur, E. I. (2006). Hepatitis C virus glycoproteins mediate low pH-dependent membrane fusion with liposomes. *J Biol Chem* 281, 3909-3917.

Lavillette, D., Morice, Y., Germanidis, G., Donot, P., Soulier, A., Pagkalos, E., Sakellariou, G., Intrator, L., Bartosch, B., Pawlotsky, J. M. & Cosset, F. L. (2005). Human serum facilitates hepatitis C virus infection, and neutralizing responses inversely correlate with viral replication kinetics at the acute phase of hepatitis C virus infection. *J Virol* 79, 6023-6034.

Lavillette, D., Pecheur, E. I., Donot, P., Fresquet, J., Molle, J., Corbau, R., Dreux, M., Penin, F. & Cosset, F. L. (2007). Characterization of fusion determinants points to the involvement of three discrete regions of both E1 and E2 glycoproteins in the membrane fusion process of hepatitis C virus. *J Virol* 81, 8752-8765.

Lechner, F., Gruener, N. H., Urbani, S., Uggeri, J., Santantonio, T., Kammer, A. R., Cerny, A., Phillips, R., Ferrari, C., Pape, G. R. & Klenerman, P. (2000a). CD8+ T lymphocyte responses are induced during acute hepatitis C virus infection but are not sustained. *Eur J Immunol* 30, 2479-2487.

Lechner, F., Wong, D. K., Dunbar, P. R., Chapman, R., Chung, R. T., Dohrenwend, P., Robbins, G., Phillips, R., Klenerman, P. & Walker, B. D. (2000b). Analysis of successful immune responses in persons infected with hepatitis C virus. *J Exp Med* 191, 1499-1512.

Levrero, M., Pollicino, T., Petersen, J., Belloni, L., Raimondo, G. & Dandri, M. (2009). Control of cccDNA function in hepatitis B virus infection. *J Hepatol* 51, 581-592.

Li, K., Foy, E., Ferreon, J. C., Nakamura, M., Ferreon, A. C., Ikeda, M., Ray, S. C., Gale, M., Jr. & Lemon, S. M. (2005a). Immune evasion by hepatitis C virus NS3/4A protease-mediated cleavage of the Toll-like receptor 3 adaptor protein TRIF. *Proc Natl Acad Sci U S A* 102, 2992-2997.

Li, X. D., Sun, L., Seth, R. B., Pineda, G. & Chen, Z. J. (2005b). Hepatitis C virus protease NS3/4A cleaves mitochondrial antiviral signaling protein off the mitochondria to evade innate immunity. *Proc Natl Acad Sci U S A* 102, 17717-17722.

Liaw, Y. F., Brunetto, M. R. & Hadziyannis, S. (2010). The natural history of chronic HBV infection and geographical differences. *Antivir Ther* 15 Suppl 3, 25-33.

Lin, W., Kim, S. S., Yeung, E., Kamegaya, Y., Blackard, J. T., Kim, K. A., Holtzman, M. J. & Chung, R. T. (2006). Hepatitis C virus core protein blocks interferon signaling by interaction with the STAT1 SH2 domain. *J Virol* 80, 9226-9235.

Lindenbach, B. D., Evans, M. J., Syder, A. J., Wolk, B., Tellinghuisen, T. L., Liu, C. C., Maruyama, T., Hynes, R. O., Burton, D. R., McKeating, J. A. & Rice, C. M. (2005). Complete replication of hepatitis C virus in cell culture. *Science* 309, 623-626.

Liu, B., Liao, J., Rao, X., Kushner, S. A., Chung, C. D., Chang, D. D. & Shuai, K. (1998). Inhibition of Stat1-mediated gene activation by PIAS1. *Proc Natl Acad Sci U S A* 95, 10626-10631.

Liu, L. Q., Ilaria, R., Jr., Kingsley, P. D., Iwama, A., van Etten, R. A., Palis, J. & Zhang, D. E. (1999). A novel ubiquitin-specific protease, UBP43, cloned from leukemia fusion protein AML1-ETO-expressing mice, functions in hematopoietic cell differentiation. *Mol Cell Biol* 19, 3029-3038.

Liu, S., Yang, W., Shen, L., Turner, J. R., Coyne, C. B. & Wang, T. (2009). Tight junction proteins claudin-1 and occludin control hepatitis C virus entry and are downregulated during infection to prevent superinfection. *J Virol* 83, 2011-2014.

Lodoen, M. B. & Lanier, L. L. (2006). Natural killer cells as an initial defense against pathogens. *Curr Opin Immunol* 18, 391-398.

Logvinoff, C., Major, M. E., Oldach, D., Heyward, S., Talal, A., Balfe, P., Feinstone, S. M., Alter, H., Rice, C. M. & McKeating, J. A. (2004). Neutralizing antibody response during acute and chronic hepatitis C virus infection. *Proc Natl Acad Sci U S A* 101, 10149-10154.

Lohmann, V., Korner, F., Koch, J., Herian, U., Theilmann, L. & Bartenschlager, R. (1999). Replication of subgenomic hepatitis C virus RNAs in a hepatoma cell line. *Science* 285, 110-113.

Longman, R. S., Talal, A. H., Jacobson, I. M., Albert, M. L. & Rice, C. M. (2004). Presence of functional dendritic cells in patients chronically infected with hepatitis C virus. *Blood* 103, 1026-1029.

Longman, R. S., Talal, A. H., Jacobson, I. M., Rice, C. M. & Albert, M. L. (2005). Normal functional capacity in circulating myeloid and plasmacytoid dendritic cells in patients with chronic hepatitis C. *J Infect Dis* 192, 497-503.

Lopes, A. R., Kellam, P., Das, A., Dunn, C., Kwan, A., Turner, J., Peppa, D., Gilson, R. J., Gehring, A., Bertoletti, A. & Maini, M. K. (2008). Bim-mediated deletion of antigen-specific CD8 T cells in patients unable to control HBV infection. *J Clin Invest* 118, 1835-1845.

Maini, M. K., Boni, C., Lee, C. K., Larrubia, J. R., Reignat, S., Ogg, G. S., King, A. S., Herberg, J., Gilson, R., Alisa, A., Williams, R., Vergani, D., Naoumov, N. V., Ferrari, C. & Bertoletti, A. (2000a). The role of virus-specific CD8(+) cells in liver damage and viral control during persistent hepatitis B virus infection. *J Exp Med* 191, 1269-1280.

Maini, M. K., Boni, C., Ogg, G. S., King, A. S., Reignat, S., Lee, C. K., Larrubia, J. R., Webster, G. J., McMichael, A. J., Ferrari, C., Williams, R., Vergani, D. & Bertoletti, A. (1999). Direct ex vivo analysis of hepatitis B virus-specific CD8(+) T cells associated with the control of infection. *Gastroenterology* 117, 1386-1396.

Maini, M. K., Reignat, S., Boni, C., Ogg, G. S., King, A. S., Malacarne, F., Webster, G. J. & Bertoletti, A. (2000b). T cell receptor usage of virus-specific CD8 cells and recognition of viral mutations during acute and persistent hepatitis B virus infection. *Eur J Immunol* 30, 3067-3078.

Maini, M. K. & Schurich, A. (2010). The molecular basis of the failed immune response in chronic HBV: therapeutic implications. *J Hepatol* 52, 616-619.

Manigold, T., Shin, E. C., Mizukoshi, E., Mihalik, K., Murthy, K. K., Rice, C. M., Piccirillo, C. A. & Rehermann, B. (2006). Foxp3+CD4+CD25+ T cells control virus-specific memory T cells in chimpanzees that recovered from hepatitis C. *Blood* 107, 4424-4432.

Manns, M. P., McHutchison, J. G., Gordon, S. C., Rustgi, V. K., Shiffman, M., Reindollar, R., Goodman, Z. D., Koury, K., Ling, M. & Albrecht, J. K. (2001). Peginterferon alfa-2b plus ribavirin compared with interferon alfa-2b plus ribavirin for initial treatment of chronic hepatitis C: a randomised trial. *Lancet* 358, 958-965.

Manns, M. P. & Rambusch, E. G. (1999). Autoimmunity and extrahepatic manifestations in hepatitis C virus infection. *J Hepatol* 31 Suppl 1, 39-42.

Marie, I., Durbin, J. E. & Levy, D. E. (1998). Differential viral induction of distinct interferon-alpha genes by positive feedback through interferon regulatory factor-7. *EMBO J* 17, 6660-6669.

Maruyama, T., Schodel, F., Iino, S., Koike, K., Yasuda, K., Peterson, D. & Milich, D. R. (1994). Distinguishing between acute and symptomatic chronic hepatitis B virus infection. *Gastroenterology* 106, 1006-1015.

McClary, H., Koch, R., Chisari, F. V. & Guidotti, L. G. (2000). Relative sensitivity of hepatitis B virus and other hepatotropic viruses to the antiviral effects of cytokines. *J Virol* 74, 2255-2264.

Meertens, L., Bertaux, C. & Dragic, T. (2006). Hepatitis C virus entry requires a critical postinternalization step and delivery to early endosomes via clathrin-coated vesicles. *J Virol* 80, 11571-11578.

Meylan, E., Curran, J., Hofmann, K., Moradpour, D., Binder, M., Bartenschlager, R. & Tschopp, J. (2005). Cardif is an adaptor protein in the RIG-I antiviral pathway and is targeted by hepatitis C virus. *Nature* 437, 1167-1172.

Milich, D. & Liang, T. J. (2003). Exploring the biological basis of hepatitis B e antigen in hepatitis B virus infection. *Hepatology* 38, 1075-1086.

Milich, D. R. & Chisari, F. V. (1982). Genetic regulation of the immune response to hepatitis B surface antigen (HBsAg). I. H-2 restriction of the murine humoral immune response to the a and d determinants of HBsAg. *J Immunol* 129, 320-325.

Milich, D. R., Jones, J. E., Hughes, J. L., Price, J., Raney, A. K. & McLachlan, A. (1990). Is a function of the secreted hepatitis B e antigen to induce immunologic tolerance in utero?. *Proc Natl Acad Sci U S A* 87, 6599-6603.

Missale, G., Bertoni, R., Lamonaca, V., Valli, A., Massari, M., Mori, C., Rumi, M. G., Houghton, M., Fiaccadori, F. & Ferrari, C. (1996). Different clinical behaviors of acute hepatitis C virus infection are associated with different vigor of the anti-viral cell-mediated immune response. *J Clin Invest* 98, 706-714.

Molina, S., Castet, V., Fournier-Wirth, C., Pichard-Garcia, L., Avner, R., Harats, D., Roitelman, J., Barbaras, R., Graber, P., Ghersa, P., Smolarsky, M., Funaro, A., Malavasi, F., Larrey, D., Coste, J., Fabre, J. M., Sa-Cunha, A. & Maurel, P. (2007). The low-density lipoprotein receptor plays a role in the infection of primary human hepatocytes by hepatitis C virus. *J Hepatol* 46, 411-419.

Monazahian, M., Bohme, I., Bonk, S., Koch, A., Scholz, C., Grethe, S. & Thomssen, R. (1999). Low density lipoprotein receptor as a candidate receptor for hepatitis C virus. *J Med Virol* 57, 223-229.

Montes-Cano, M. A., Caro-Oleas, J. L., Romero-Gomez, M., Diago, M., Andrade, R., Carmona, I., Aguilar Reina, J., Nunez-Roldan, A. & Gonzalez-Escribano, M. F. (2005). HLA-C and KIR genes in hepatitis C virus infection. *Hum Immunol* 66, 1106-1109.

Moradpour, D., Brass, V., Bieck, E., Friebe, P., Gosert, R., Blum, H. E., Bartenschlager, R., Penin, F. & Lohmann, V. (2004). Membrane association of the RNA-dependent

RNA polymerase is essential for hepatitis C virus RNA replication. *J Virol* 78, 13278-13284.

Moretta, L., Bottino, C., Pende, D., Vitale, M., Mingari, M. C. & Moretta, A. (2005). Human natural killer cells: Molecular mechanisms controlling NK cell activation and tumor cell lysis. *Immunol Lett* 100, 7-13.

Nakamoto, N., Cho, H., Shaked, A., Olthoff, K., Valiga, M. E., Kaminski, M., Gostick, E., Price, D. A., Freeman, G. J., Wherry, E. J. & Chang, K. M. (2009). Synergistic reversal of intrahepatic HCV-specific CD8 T cell exhaustion by combined PD-1/CTLA-4 blockade. *PLoS Pathog* 5, e1000313.

Nakamoto, N., Kaplan, D. E., Coleclough, J., Li, Y., Valiga, M. E., Kaminski, M., Shaked, A., Olthoff, K., Gostick, E., Price, D. A., Freeman, G. J., Wherry, E. J. & Chang, K. M. (2008). Functional restoration of HCV-specific CD8 T cells by PD-1 blockade is defined by PD-1 expression and compartmentalization. *Gastroenterology* 134, 1927-1937, 1937 e1921-1922.

Nascimbeni, M., Mizukoshi, E., Bosmann, M., Major, M. E., Mihalik, K., Rice, C. M., Feinstone, S. M. & Rehermann, B. (2003). Kinetics of CD4+ and CD8+ memory T-cell responses during hepatitis C virus rechallenge of previously recovered chimpanzees. *J Virol* 77, 4781-4793.

Neumann-Haefelin, C., McKiernan, S., Ward, S., Viazov, S., Spangenberg, H. C., Killinger, T., Baumert, T. F., Nazarova, N., Sheridan, I., Pybus, O., von Weizsacker, F., Roggendorf, M., Kelleher, D., Klenerman, P., Blum, H. E. & Thimme, R. (2006). Dominant influence of an HLA-B27 restricted CD8+ T cell response in mediating HCV clearance and evolution. *Hepatology* 43, 563-572.

Nowak, M. A. & Bangham, C. R. (1996). Population dynamics of immune responses to persistent viruses. *Science* 272, 74-79.

Oliviero, B., Varchetta, S., Paudice, E., Michelone, G., Zaramella, M., Mavilio, D., De Filippi, F., Bruno, S. & Mondelli, M. U. (2009). Natural killer cell functional dichotomy in chronic hepatitis B and chronic hepatitis C virus infections. *Gastroenterology* 137, 1151-1160, 1160 e1151-1157.

Paladino, N., Flores, A. C., Marcos, C. Y., Fainboim, H., Theiler, G., Arruvito, L., Williams, F., Middleton, D. & Fainboim, L. (2007). Increased frequencies of activating natural killer receptors are associated with liver injury in individuals who do not eliminate hepatitis C virus. *Tissue Antigens* 69 Suppl 1, 109-111.

Pavio, N. & Lai, M. M. (2003). The hepatitis C virus persistence: how to evade the immune system? *J Biosci* 28, 287-304.

Pawlotsky, J. M. (2004). Pathophysiology of hepatitis C virus infection and related liver disease. *Trends Microbiol* 12, 96-102.

Penna, A., Artini, M., Cavalli, A., Levrero, M., Bertoletti, A., Pilli, M., Chisari, F. V., Rehermann, B., Del Prete, G., Fiaccadori, F. & Ferrari, C. (1996). Long-lasting memory T cell responses following self-limited acute hepatitis B. *J Clin Invest* 98, 1185-1194.

Penna, A., Pilli, M., Zerbini, A., Orlandini, A., Mezzadri, S., Sacchelli, L., Missale, G. & Ferrari, C. (2007). Dysfunction and functional restoration of HCV-specific CD8 responses in chronic hepatitis C virus infection. *Hepatology* 45, 588-601.

Perrillo, R., Hou, J., Papatheodoridis, G. & Manns, M. (2010). Patient management and clinical decision making in HBV--aims of therapy and what we can achieve. *Antivir Ther* 15 Suppl 3, 45-51.

Pestka, J. M., Zeisel, M. B., Blaser, E., Schurmann, P., Bartosch, B., Cosset, F. L., Patel, A. H., Meisel, H., Baumert, J., Viazov, S., Rispeter, K., Blum, H. E., Roggendorf, M. & Baumert, T. F. (2007). Rapid induction of virus-neutralizing antibodies and viral clearance in a single-source outbreak of hepatitis C. *Proc Natl Acad Sci U S A* 104, 6025-6030.

Piazzolla, G., Tortorella, C., Schiraldi, O. & Antonaci, S. (2000). Relationship between interferon-gamma, interleukin-10, and interleukin-12 production in chronic hepatitis C and in vitro effects of interferon-alpha. *J Clin Immunol* 20, 54-61.

Pileri, P., Uematsu, Y., Campagnoli, S., Galli, G., Falugi, F., Petracca, R., Weiner, A. J., Houghton, M., Rosa, D., Grandi, G. & Abrignani, S. (1998). Binding of hepatitis C virus to CD81. *Science* 282, 938-941.

Pilli, M., Zerbini, A., Penna, A., Orlandini, A., Lukasiewicz, E., Pawlotsky, J. M., Zeuzem, S., Schalm, S. W., von Wagner, M., Germanidis, G., Lurie, Y., Esteban, J. I., Haagmans, B. L., Hezode, C., Lagging, M., Negro, F., Homburger, Y., Neumann, A. U., Ferrari, C. & Missale, G. (2007). HCV-specific T-cell response in relation to viral kinetics and treatment outcome (DITTO-HCV project). *Gastroenterology* 133, 1132-1143.

Ploss, A., Evans, M. J., Gaysinskaya, V. A., Panis, M., You, H., de Jong, Y. P. & Rice, C. M. (2009). Human occludin is a hepatitis C virus entry factor required for infection of mouse cells. *Nature* 457, 882-886.

Polyak, S. J., Khabar, K. S., Paschal, D. M., Ezelle, H. J., Duverlie, G., Barber, G. N., Levy, D. E., Mukaida, N. & Gretch, D. R. (2001). Hepatitis C virus nonstructural 5A protein induces interleukin-8, leading to partial inhibition of the interferon-induced antiviral response. *J Virol* 75, 6095-6106.

Poordad, F., McCone, J., Jr., Bacon, B. R., Bruno, S., Manns, M. P., Sulkowski, M. S., Jacobson, I. M., Reddy, K. R., Goodman, Z. D., Boparai, N., DiNubile, M. J., Sniukiene, V., Brass, C. A., Albrecht, J. K. & Bronowicki, J. P. (2011). Boceprevir for untreated chronic HCV genotype 1 infection. *N Engl J Med* 364, 1195-1206.

Racanelli, V., Frassanito, M. A., Leone, P., Galiano, M., De Re, V., Silvestris, F. & Dammacco, F. (2006). Antibody production and in vitro behavior of CD27-defined B-cell subsets: persistent hepatitis C virus infection changes the rules. *J Virol* 80, 3923-3934.

Racanelli, V. & Rehermann, B. (2006). The liver as an immunological organ. *Hepatology* 43, S54-62.

Radziewicz, H., Ibegbu, C. C., Fernandez, M. L., Workowski, K. A., Obideen, K., Wehbi, M., Hanson, H. L., Steinberg, J. P., Masopust, D., Wherry, E. J., Altman, J. D., Rouse, B. T., Freeman, G. J., Ahmed, R. & Grakoui, A. (2007). Liver-infiltrating lymphocytes in chronic human hepatitis C virus infection display an exhausted phenotype with high levels of PD-1 and low levels of CD127 expression. *J Virol* 81, 2545-2553.

Rahman, F., Heller, T., Sobao, Y., Mizukoshi, E., Nascimbeni, M., Alter, H., Herrine, S., Hoofnagle, J., Liang, T. J. & Rehermann, B. (2004). Effects of antiviral therapy on the cellular immune response in acute hepatitis C. *Hepatology* 40, 87-97.

Rauch, A., Laird, R., McKinnon, E., Telenti, A., Furrer, H., Weber, R., Smillie, D. & Gaudieri, S. (2007). Influence of inhibitory killer immunoglobulin-like receptors and their

HLA-C ligands on resolving hepatitis C virus infection. *Tissue Antigens* 69 Suppl 1, 237-240.

Ray, S. C., Fanning, L., Wang, X. H., Netski, D. M., Kenny-Walsh, E. & Thomas, D. L. (2005). Divergent and convergent evolution after a common-source outbreak of hepatitis C virus. *J Exp Med* 201, 1753-1759.

Rehermann, B. (2009). Hepatitis C virus versus innate and adaptive immune responses: a tale of coevolution and coexistence. *J Clin Invest* 119, 1745-1754.

Rehermann, B., Ferrari, C., Pasquinelli, C. & Chisari, F. V. (1996). The hepatitis B virus persists for decades after patients' recovery from acute viral hepatitis despite active maintenance of a cytotoxic T-lymphocyte response. *Nat Med* 2, 1104-1108.

Riordan, S. M., Skinner, N., Kurtovic, J., Locarnini, S. & Visvanathan, K. (2006). Reduced expression of toll-like receptor 2 on peripheral monocytes in patients with chronic hepatitis B. *Clin Vaccine Immunol* 13, 972-974.

Rong, L., Dahari, H., Ribeiro, R. M. & Perelson, A. S. (2010). Rapid emergence of protease inhibitor resistance in hepatitis C virus. *Sci Transl Med* 2, 30ra32.

Rushbrook, S. M., Ward, S. M., Unitt, E., Vowler, S. L., Lucas, M., Klenerman, P. & Alexander, G. J. (2005). Regulatory T cells suppress in vitro proliferation of virus-specific CD8+ T cells during persistent hepatitis C virus infection. *J Virol* 79, 7852-7859.

Rutebemberwa, A., Ray, S. C., Astemborski, J., Levine, J., Liu, L., Dowd, K. A., Clute, S., Wang, C., Korman, A., Sette, A., Sidney, J., Pardoll, D. M. & Cox, A. L. (2008). High-programmed death-1 levels on hepatitis C virus-specific T cells during acute infection are associated with viral persistence and require preservation of cognate antigen during chronic infection. *J Immunol* 181, 8215-8225.

Saito, T., Owen, D. M., Jiang, F., Marcotrigiano, J. & Gale, M., Jr. (2008). Innate immunity induced by composition-dependent RIG-I recognition of hepatitis C virus RNA. *Nature* 454, 523-527.

Sakamoto, H., Kinjyo, I. & Yoshimura, A. (2000). The janus kinase inhibitor, Jab/SOCS-1, is an interferon-gamma inducible gene and determines the sensitivity to interferons. *Leuk Lymphoma* 38, 49-58.

Samuel, C. E. (2001). Antiviral actions of interferons. *Clin Microbiol Rev* 14, 778-809, table of contents.

Sarobe, P., Lasarte, J. J., Zabaleta, A., Arribillaga, L., Arina, A., Melero, I., Borras-Cuesta, F. & Prieto, J. (2003). Hepatitis C virus structural proteins impair dendritic cell maturation and inhibit in vivo induction of cellular immune responses. *J Virol* 77, 10862-10871.

Sato, M., Suemori, H., Hata, N., Asagiri, M., Ogasawara, K., Nakao, K., Nakaya, T., Katsuki, M., Noguchi, S., Tanaka, N. & Taniguchi, T. (2000). Distinct and essential roles of transcription factors IRF-3 and IRF-7 in response to viruses for IFN-alpha/beta gene induction. *Immunity* 13, 539-548.

Saunier, B., Triyatni, M., Ulianich, L., Maruvada, P., Yen, P. & Kohn, L. D. (2003). Role of the asialoglycoprotein receptor in binding and entry of hepatitis C virus structural proteins in cultured human hepatocytes. *J Virol* 77, 546-559.

Scarselli, E., Ansuini, H., Cerino, R., Roccasecca, R. M., Acali, S., Filocamo, G., Traboni, C., Nicosia, A., Cortese, R. & Vitelli, A. (2002). The human scavenger receptor class B type I is a novel candidate receptor for the hepatitis C virus. *EMBO J* 21, 5017-5025.

Seifert, U., Liermann, H., Racanelli, V., Halenius, A., Wiese, M., Wedemeyer, H., Ruppert, T., Rispeter, K., Henklein, P., Sijts, A., Hengel, H., Kloetzel, P. M. & Rehermann, B. (2004). Hepatitis C virus mutation affects proteasomal epitope processing. *J Clin Invest* 114, 250-259.

Semmo, N., Lucas, M., Krashias, G., Lauer, G., Chapel, H. & Klenerman, P. (2006). Maintenance of HCV-specific T-cell responses in antibody-deficient patients a decade after early therapy. *Blood* 107, 4570-4571.

Sharpe, A. H., Wherry, E. J., Ahmed, R. & Freeman, G. J. (2007). The function of programmed cell death 1 and its ligands in regulating autoimmunity and infection. *Nat Immunol* 8, 239-245.

Shevach, E. M. (2009). Mechanisms of foxp3+ T regulatory cell-mediated suppression. *Immunity* 30, 636-645.

Shields, P. L., Morland, C. M., Salmon, M., Qin, S., Hubscher, S. G. & Adams, D. H. (1999). Chemokine and chemokine receptor interactions provide a mechanism for selective T cell recruitment to specific liver compartments within hepatitis C-infected liver. *J Immunol* 163, 6236-6243.

Shin, E. C., Seifert, U., Kato, T., Rice, C. M., Feinstone, S. M., Kloetzel, P. M. & Rehermann, B. (2006). Virus-induced type I IFN stimulates generation of immunoproteasomes at the site of infection. *J Clin Invest* 116, 3006-3014.

Sillanpaa, M., Kaukinen, P., Melen, K. & Julkunen, I. (2008). Hepatitis C virus proteins interfere with the activation of chemokine gene promoters and downregulate chemokine gene expression. *J Gen Virol* 89, 432-443.

Smyk-Pearson, S., Tester, I. A., Klarquist, J., Palmer, B. E., Pawlotsky, J. M., Golden-Mason, L. & Rosen, H. R. (2008). Spontaneous recovery in acute human hepatitis C virus infection: functional T-cell thresholds and relative importance of CD4 help. *J Virol* 82, 1827-1837.

Sprengers, D., van der Molen, R. G., Binda, R., Kusters, J. G., de Man, R. A., Niesters, H. G., Schalm, S. W. & Janssen, H. L. (2007). In vivo immunization in combination with peg-interferon for chronic hepatitis B virus infection. *J Viral Hepat* 14, 743-749.

Sprengers, D., van der Molen, R. G., Kusters, J. G., Kwekkeboom, J., van der Laan, L. J., Niesters, H. G., Kuipers, E. J., De Man, R. A., Schalm, S. W. & Janssen, H. L. (2005). Flow cytometry of fine-needle-aspiration biopsies: a new method to monitor the intrahepatic immunological environment in chronic viral hepatitis. *J Viral Hepat* 12, 507-512.

Springer, T. A. (1994). Traffic signals for lymphocyte recirculation and leukocyte emigration: the multistep paradigm. *Cell* 76, 301-314.

Stegmann, K. A., Bjorkstrom, N. K., Veber, H., Ciesek, S., Riese, P., Wiegand, J., Hadem, J., Suneetha, P. V., Jaroszewicz, J., Wang, C., Schlaphoff, V., Fytili, P., Cornberg, M., Manns, M. P., Geffers, R., Pietschmann, T., Guzman, C. A., Ljunggren, H. G. & Wedemeyer, H. (2010). Interferon-alpha-induced TRAIL on natural killer cells is associated with control of hepatitis C virus infection. *Gastroenterology* 138, 1885-1897.

Steinman, R. M., Hawiger, D. & Nussenzweig, M. C. (2003). Tolerogenic dendritic cells. *Annu Rev Immunol* 21, 685-711.

Stoop, J. N., van der Molen, R. G., Kuipers, E. J., Kusters, J. G. & Janssen, H. L. (2007). Inhibition of viral replication reduces regulatory T cells and enhances the antiviral immune response in chronic hepatitis B. *Virology* 361, 141-148.

Sugimoto, K., Ikeda, F., Stadanlick, J., Nunes, F. A., Alter, H. J. & Chang, K. M. (2003). Suppression of HCV-specific T cells without differential hierarchy demonstrated ex vivo in persistent HCV infection. *Hepatology* 38, 1437-1448.

Szabo, G. & Dolganiuc, A. (2005). Subversion of plasmacytoid and myeloid dendritic cell functions in chronic HCV infection. *Immunobiology* 210, 237-247.

Tan, A. T., Koh, S., Goh, W., Zhe, H. Y., Gehring, A. J., Lim, S. G. & Bertoletti, A. (2010). A longitudinal analysis of innate and adaptive immune profile during hepatic flares in chronic hepatitis B. *J Hepatol* 52, 330-339.

Taylor, D. R., Shi, S. T., Romano, P. R., Barber, G. N. & Lai, M. M. (1999). Inhibition of the interferon-inducible protein kinase PKR by HCV E2 protein. *Science* 285, 107-110.

Tester, I., Smyk-Pearson, S., Wang, P., Wertheimer, A., Yao, E., Lewinsohn, D. M., Tavis, J. E. & Rosen, H. R. (2005). Immune evasion versus recovery after acute hepatitis C virus infection from a shared source. *J Exp Med* 201, 1725-1731.

Thimme, R., Bukh, J., Spangenberg, H. C., Wieland, S., Pemberton, J., Steiger, C., Govindarajan, S., Purcell, R. H. & Chisari, F. V. (2002). Viral and immunological determinants of hepatitis C virus clearance, persistence, and disease. *Proc Natl Acad Sci U S A* 99, 15661-15668.

Thimme, R., Lohmann, V. & Weber, F. (2006). A target on the move: innate and adaptive immune escape strategies of hepatitis C virus. *Antiviral Res* 69, 129-141.

Thimme, R., Oldach, D., Chang, K. M., Steiger, C., Ray, S. C. & Chisari, F. V. (2001). Determinants of viral clearance and persistence during acute hepatitis C virus infection. *J Exp Med* 194, 1395-1406.

Timm, J., Lauer, G. M., Kavanagh, D. G., Sheridan, I., Kim, A. Y., Lucas, M., Pillay, T., Ouchi, K., Reyor, L. L., Schulze zur Wiesch, J., Gandhi, R. T., Chung, R. T., Bhardwaj, N., Klenerman, P., Walker, B. D. & Allen, T. M. (2004). CD8 epitope escape and reversion in acute HCV infection. *J Exp Med* 200, 1593-1604.

Trautmann, L., Janbazian, L., Chomont, N., Said, E. A., Gimmig, S., Bessette, B., Boulassel, M. R., Delwart, E., Sepulveda, H., Balderas, R. S., Routy, J. P., Haddad, E. K. & Sekaly, R. P. (2006). Upregulation of PD-1 expression on HIV-specific CD8+ T cells leads to reversible immune dysfunction. *Nat Med* 12, 1198-1202.

Tscherne, D. M., Jones, C. T., Evans, M. J., Lindenbach, B. D., McKeating, J. A. & Rice, C. M. (2006). Time- and temperature-dependent activation of hepatitis C virus for low-pH-triggered entry. *J Virol* 80, 1734-1741.

Tsukuma, H., Hiyama, T., Tanaka, S., Nakao, M., Yabuuchi, T., Kitamura, T., Nakanishi, K., Fujimoto, I., Inoue, A., Yamazaki, H. & et al. (1993). Risk factors for hepatocellular carcinoma among patients with chronic liver disease. *N Engl J Med* 328, 1797-1801.

Urban, S., Schulze, A., Dandri, M. & Petersen, J. (2010). The replication cycle of hepatitis B virus. *J Hepatol* 52, 282-284.

Urbani, S., Amadei, B., Fisicaro, P., Tola, D., Orlandini, A., Sacchelli, L., Mori, C., Missale, G. & Ferrari, C. (2006a). Outcome of acute hepatitis C is related to virus-specific CD4 function and maturation of antiviral memory CD8 responses. *Hepatology* 44, 126-139.

Urbani, S., Amadei, B., Tola, D., Massari, M., Schivazappa, S., Missale, G. & Ferrari, C. (2006b). PD-1 expression in acute hepatitis C virus (HCV) infection is associated with HCV-specific CD8 exhaustion. *J Virol* 80, 11398-11403.

Veerapu, N. S., Raghuraman, S., Liang, T. J., Heller, T. & Rehermann, B. (2011). Sporadic reappearance of minute amounts of hepatitis C virus RNA after successful therapy stimulates cellular immune responses. *Gastroenterology* 140, 676-685 e671.

Visvanathan, K., Skinner, N. A., Thompson, A. J., Riordan, S. M., Sozzi, V., Edwards, R., Rodgers, S., Kurtovic, J., Chang, J., Lewin, S., Desmond, P. & Locarnini, S. (2007). Regulation of Toll-like receptor-2 expression in chronic hepatitis B by the precore protein. *Hepatology* 45, 102-110.

von Hahn, T., Yoon, J. C., Alter, H., Rice, C. M., Rehermann, B., Balfe, P. & McKeating, J. A. (2007). Hepatitis C virus continuously escapes from neutralizing antibody and T-cell responses during chronic infection in vivo. *Gastroenterology* 132, 667-678.

Wakita, T., Pietschmann, T., Kato, T., Date, T., Miyamoto, M., Zhao, Z., Murthy, K., Habermann, A., Krausslich, H. G., Mizokami, M., Bartenschlager, R. & Liang, T. J. (2005). Production of infectious hepatitis C virus in tissue culture from a cloned viral genome. *Nat Med* 11, 791-796.

Wang, J., Zhao, J. H., Wang, P. P. & Xiang, G. J. (2008). Expression of CXC chemokine IP-10 in patients with chronic hepatitis B. *Hepatobiliary Pancreat Dis Int* 7, 45-50.

Webster, G. J., Reignat, S., Brown, D., Ogg, G. S., Jones, L., Seneviratne, S. L., Williams, R., Dusheiko, G. & Bertoletti, A. (2004). Longitudinal analysis of CD8+ T cells specific for structural and nonstructural hepatitis B virus proteins in patients with chronic hepatitis B: implications for immunotherapy. *J Virol* 78, 5707-5719.

Webster, G. J., Reignat, S., Maini, M. K., Whalley, S. A., Ogg, G. S., King, A., Brown, D., Amlot, P. L., Williams, R., Vergani, D., Dusheiko, G. M. & Bertoletti, A. (2000). Incubation phase of acute hepatitis B in man: dynamic of cellular immune mechanisms. *Hepatology* 32, 1117-1124.

Wieland, S., Thimme, R., Purcell, R. H. & Chisari, F. V. (2004). Genomic analysis of the host response to hepatitis B virus infection. *Proc Natl Acad Sci U S A* 101, 6669-6674.

Wieland, S. F. & Chisari, F. V. (2005). Stealth and cunning: hepatitis B and hepatitis C viruses. *J Virol* 79, 9369-9380.

Wieland, S. F., Guidotti, L. G. & Chisari, F. V. (2000). Intrahepatic induction of alpha/beta interferon eliminates viral RNA-containing capsids in hepatitis B virus transgenic mice. *J Virol* 74, 4165-4173.

Wu, J., Meng, Z., Jiang, M., Pei, R., Trippler, M., Broering, R., Bucchi, A., Sowa, J. P., Dittmer, U., Yang, D., Roggendorf, M., Gerken, G., Lu, M. & Schlaak, J. F. (2009). Hepatitis B virus suppresses toll-like receptor-mediated innate immune responses in murine parenchymal and nonparenchymal liver cells. *Hepatology* 49, 1132-1140.

Wu, J. F., Wu, T. C., Chen, C. H., Ni, Y. H., Chen, H. L., Hsu, H. Y. & Chang, M. H. (2010). Serum levels of interleukin-10 and interleukin-12 predict early, spontaneous hepatitis B virus e antigen seroconversion. *Gastroenterology* 138, 165-172 e161-163.

Wunschmann, S., Medh, J. D., Klinzmann, D., Schmidt, W. N. & Stapleton, J. T. (2000). Characterization of hepatitis C virus (HCV) and HCV E2 interactions with CD81 and the low-density lipoprotein receptor. *J Virol* 74, 10055-10062.

Xie, Q., Shen, H. C., Jia, N. N., Wang, H., Lin, L. Y., An, B. Y., Gui, H. L., Guo, S. M., Cai, W., Yu, H., Guo, Q. & Bao, S. (2009). Patients with chronic hepatitis B infection display deficiency of plasmacytoid dendritic cells with reduced expression of TLR9. *Microbes Infect* 11, 515-523.

Xu, L. G., Wang, Y. Y., Han, K. J., Li, L. Y., Zhai, Z. & Shu, H. B. (2005). VISA is an adapter protein required for virus-triggered IFN-beta signaling. *Mol Cell* 19, 727-740.

Yerly, D., Heckerman, D., Allen, T. M., Chisholm, J. V., 3rd, Faircloth, K., Linde, C. H., Frahm, N., Timm, J., Pichler, W. J., Cerny, A. & Brander, C. (2008). Increased cytotoxic T-lymphocyte epitope variant cross-recognition and functional avidity are associated with hepatitis C virus clearance. *J Virol* 82, 3147-3153.

Zeisel, M. B., Cosset, F. L. & Baumert, T. F. (2008). Host neutralizing responses and pathogenesis of hepatitis C virus infection. *Hepatology* 48, 299-307.

Zerbini, A., Pilli, M., Boni, C., Fisicaro, P., Penna, A., Di Vincenzo, P., Giuberti, T., Orlandini, A., Raffa, G., Pollicino, T., Raimondo, G., Ferrari, C. & Missale, G. (2008). The characteristics of the cell-mediated immune response identify different profiles of occult hepatitis B virus infection. *Gastroenterology* 134, 1470-1481.

Zhang, J. Y., Song, C. H., Shi, F., Zhang, Z., Fu, J. L. & Wang, F. S. (2010). Decreased ratio of Treg cells to Th17 cells correlates with HBV DNA suppression in chronic hepatitis B patients undergoing entecavir treatment. *PLoS One* 5, e13869.

Zhang, P., Zhong, L., Struble, E. B., Watanabe, H., Kachko, A., Mihalik, K., Virata-Theimer, M. L., Alter, H. J., Feinstone, S. & Major, M. (2009). Depletion of interfering antibodies in chronic hepatitis C patients and vaccinated chimpanzees reveals broad cross-genotype neutralizing activity. *Proc Natl Acad Sci U S A* 106, 7537-7541.

Zhao, C., Beaudenon, S. L., Kelley, M. L., Waddell, M. B., Yuan, W., Schulman, B. A., Huibregtse, J. M. & Krug, R. M. (2004). The UbcH8 ubiquitin E2 enzyme is also the E2 enzyme for ISG15, an IFN-alpha/beta-induced ubiquitin-like protein. *Proc Natl Acad Sci U S A* 101, 7578-7582.

Zhong, J., Gastaminza, P., Cheng, G., Kapadia, S., Kato, T., Burton, D. R., Wieland, S. F., Uprichard, S. L., Wakita, T. & Chisari, F. V. (2005). Robust hepatitis C virus infection in vitro. *Proc Natl Acad Sci U S A* 102, 9294-9299.

2

Toll Like Receptors in Chronic Viral Hepatitis – Friend and Foe

Ruth Broering, Mengji Lu and Joerg F. Schlaak
University Hospital of Essen
Germany

1. Introduction

Chronic viral hepatitis caused by Hepatitis B virus (HBV), Hepatitis C virus (HCV) and Hepatitis D virus (HDV) infection is among the most frequent causes for liver related morbidity and mortality worldwide. In recent years, it has become clear that not only the adaptive but also the innate immune system is involved in the pathogenesis of these infections. The innate immune system represents the initial line of host defense against invading pathogens. Germline-encoded pathogen recognition receptors (PRR), that are able to recognize specific structures of microorganisms, are an important component of this system. Amongst these, Toll like receptors (TLR) are a family of PRR perceiving a wide range of microorganisms, including bacteria, fungi, protozoa and viruses. Hepatitis viruses have evolved evading strategies to subvert the innate immune system of the liver which is of relevance for understanding the mechanisms that lead to chronicity of these infections and to develop novel therapeutic approaches based on these findings. Thus, recent studies suggested that TLR-based therapies may represent a promising approach in the treatment in viral hepatitis. This chapter focuses on the role of local innate immunity of the liver in the pathogenesis of chronic viral hepatitis.

2. Innate immunity

It has been suggested that the innate immune system is of particular relevance in the early phase of viral and bacterial infections (Fearon and Locksley, 1996). PRR become activated immediately after exposure to infectious agents and activation of downstream signaling pathways leads to the expression of effector molecules that limit microbial replication (Biron, 1998; Epstein *et al.* 1996). PRR sense evolutionary highly conserved structures, so-called pathogen-associated molecular patterns (PAMPs). Within this process the TLR system is one of the main players (Medzhitov & Janeway, Jr., 2000; Medzhitov, 2001).

2.1 Toll like receptor system

Activation of the TLR system leads to the expression of pro-inflammatory (IL-6, IL-12, TNF-α,…) as well as anti-inflammatory cytokines (IL-10,…) by responsive cell types. TLR7, -8 and -9 additionally initiate Interferon-α (IFN-α) expression after binding of their specific ligands. Stimulation of TLR3 and -4 results in expression of IFN-β as well as immunoregulatory cytokines (Akira *et al.* 2006; Takeda & Akira, 2005).

TLRs are associated with cellular membranes and have a highly conserved cytosolic domain with similarity to the Interleukin-1 receptor and are therefore called Toll/IL-1 receptor (TIR). Binding of a specific pathogen-associated molecular pattern (PAMP) to these receptors leads to recruitment and activation of adapter molecules. All TLRs except TLR3 are able to activate the myeloid differentiation primary response gene 88 (MyD88). TLR2 and -4 integrate the TIR domain containing adapter protein (TIRAP) to active MyD88. MyD88-dependent signaling further involves Interleukin-1 receptor associated kinases 1 (IRAK1) and -4 (IRAK4) and Tumor necrosis factor (TNF) receptor associated factor 6 (TRAF6) to dissociate the Nuclear factor Kappa B (NFκB)-Inhibitor IκB. This is followed by translocation of NFκB into the nucleus and transcription of immunoregulatory genes (Takeda & Akira, 2005). MyD88 signaling additionally activates mitogen-activated protein kinases (MAPKs) which further activate AP-1 signaling resulting in cytokine expression. MyD88 signaling of endosomally located TLR7, -8 and -9 additionally promotes activation of Interferon regulatory factor 7 (IRF-7) which initiates the expression of IFN-α (Honda & Taniguchi, 2006).

TLR3 signaling is MyD88 independent. Activation of the TIR domain containing adaptor inducing IFN-β (TRIF) results in phosphorylation of IRF-3 followed by induction of IFN-β expression. TRIF additionally mediates activation of TRAF6 leading to translocation of NFκB as described before. TLR4 activates the toll-interleukin 1 receptor domain containing adaptor protein (TIRAP) to activate MyD88-dependent signaling as well as the TRIF-related adaptor molecule (TRAM) to enable TRIF dependent induction of IFN-β (Akira & Takeda, 2004; Honda & Taniguchi, 2006; Takeda and Akira, 2005) (Figure 1).

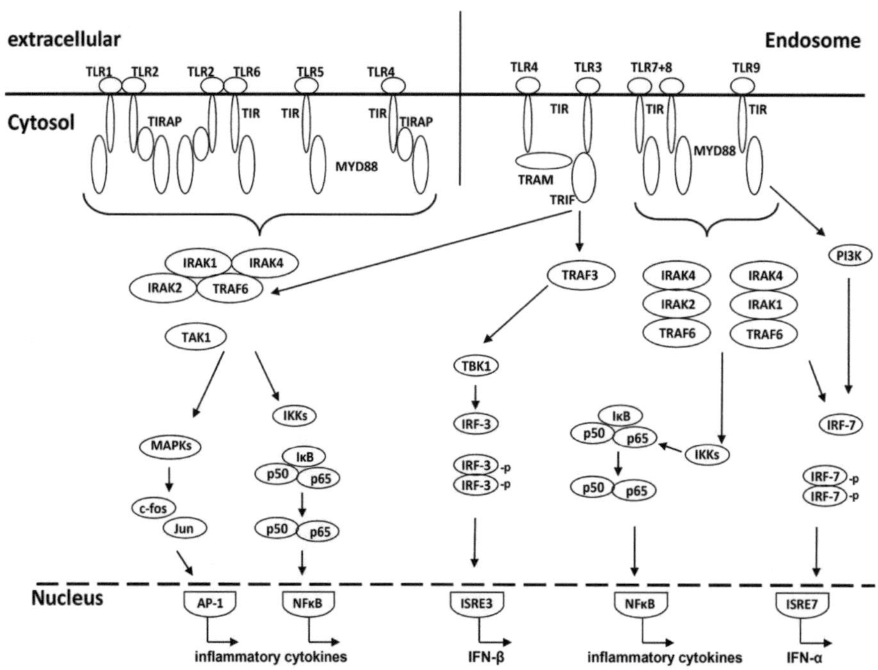

Fig. 1. Toll like receptor signaling
Activation of Toll like receptors leads to recruitment of the adaptor molecules MYD88, TIRAP, TRIF and TRAM. Downstream signaling involves TAK1, MAPKs, TRAF3, TBK1 and IKKs leading to nuclear translocation of transcriptions factors (AP-1, NFκB, IRF-3 or IRF-7) and subsequent transcription of inflammatory genes.

2.2 Local immune system of the liver

The liver represents an immunological organ in which blood from the gastrointestinal tract, enriched with nutrients and antigens, flows through sinusoids in close contact to antigen-presenting cells (APC) and lymphocytes (Figure 2). Physiological functions of the liver include protein synthesis and metabolism as well as removal of pathogens and antigens from the blood. This necessitates a locally regulated immune system. Efficient elimination of pathogenic microorganisms derived from the gastrointestinal tract must be accompanied by tolerance induction for a large number of harmless antigens to avoid unnecessary damage of hepatocytes that represent two third of the total liver cell population (Knolle & Gerken, 2000). The remaining cells consist of non-parenchymal liver cells (NPC) including Kupffer cells (KC), liver sinusoidal endothelial cells (LSEC), stellate cells, dendritic cells (DC) and intrahepatic lymphocytes.

It has been proposed that the liver is an organ of tolerance induction rather than induction of immunity. Therefore, the different types of APC may contribute in different ways to reach homeostasis of the local microenvironment (Racanelli & Rehermann, 2006). LSECs represent about 50% of the NPCs and form a fenestrated monolayer separating hepatocytes from the blood stream. LSECs are able to perform receptor-mediated endocytosis or phagocytosis with comparable efficacy as DCs. Processed peptides are loaded onto the major histocompatibility complex (MHC) class I and II molecules and are presented to passing lymphocytes. KCs represent approximately 20% of the NPC population of the liver, located in the hepatic sinusoids, where they are in close contact to the blood and passing lymphocytes. This exposed location enables Kupffer cells to take up antigens or debris from the blood stream and to induce inflammation or maintenance of tolerance (Sun *et al.* 2003).

2.3 The role of liver cells as part of the local innate immunity

TLR have recently been recognized to play an important role in the pathogenesis of chronic hepatitis. Activation of TLR signaling pathways results in an antiviral state of liver cells, thereby offering the possibility for the development of novel therapeutic strategies. Hepatocytes express TLRs and are able to respond to stimulation with TLR ligands. The expression of TLRs was demonstrated for primary human and murine hepatocytes as well as hepatoma cell lines including HepG2 and Huh7. The functionality of the TLR pathways in these cell systems was shown by analysis of cellular responses to various TLR ligands (Preiss *et al.* 2008; Thompson *et al.* 2009; Xia *et al.* 2008; Wu *et al.* 2007; Zhang *et al.* 2009; Broering *et al.* 2008).

Non-parenchymal liver cells; Kupffer cells; sinusoidal endothelial cells and hepatic stellate cells are important players to mount local innate and adaptive immune responses in the liver (Kimura *et al.* 2002; Knolle & Gerken, 2000). Studies regarding the diversification of TLR signaling pathways in NPC revealed that KC respond to all TLR ligands by producing TNF-α or IL-6. Only TLR3 and TLR4 activation leads to expression of IFN-β in KC. In addition, TLR1 and -8 ligands significantly upregulate MHC class II and costimulatory molecules. For TLR8-activated KC, high levels of T cell proliferation and IFN-γ production could be shown in mixed lymphocyte reactions (MLR). Similarly, LSEC respond to TLR3 ligands by producing IFN-β, to TLR1-4, -6 and TLR8-9 ligands by producing TNF-α, and to TLR3 and -4 ligands by producing IL-6. Interestingly, LSEC failed to stimulate allogeneic T cells in MLR despite significant upregulation of MHC class II and costimulatory molecules in response to TLR8 ligands (Wu *et al.* 2009). Taken together, NPC display a restricted TLR-mediated activation profile when compared to 'classical' APCs which may also explain, at least in part, their tolerogenic function in the liver.

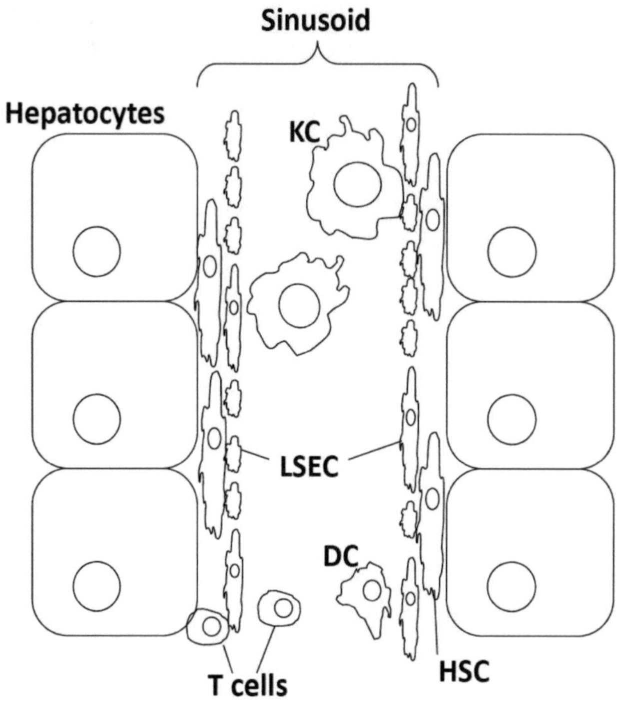

Fig. 2. Cell populations of the hepatic microenvironment
The hepatocytes are lined by the liver sinusoid endothelial cells (LSEC), preventing direct cell to cell contact to passing leucocytes, Kupffer cells (KC), dendritic cells (DC) or lymphocytes (T cells). Hepatic stellate cells (HSC) are located in the Space of Dissé between LSECs and hepatocytes.

3. Chronic viral hepatitis

Currently, five different human hepatitis viruses have been characterized: Hepatitis A virus (HAV), hepatitis B virus (HBV), hepatitis C virus (HCV), hepatitis D virus (HDV) and hepatitis E virus (HEV). HAV is a single-stranded, unenveloped RNA virus encoding for a single polyprotein. HBV is a virus with a partially double stranded DNA genome that replicates through RNA intermediates. HCV is a single-stranded RNA virus coding for a polyprotein, which is cleaved into a capsid protein, two envelope proteins and 6 non-structural proteins. HDV is a defective RNA virus, similar to viroids, that only encodes the capsid antigen (delta antigen) and is dependent upon the HBV coinfection, in particular the surface protein (HBsAg), for production of infectious virus particles. HEV is a labile RNA virus, unrelated to the other known hepatitis viruses. Chronic infections of hepatitis viruses, that are caused by HBV, HCV and HDV in immunocompetent patients, are frequently associated with progression of fibrosis and the development of liver cirrhosis and primary hepatocellular carcinoma (Hayashi & Zeldis, 1993; Perrault & Pecheur, 2009; Wedemeyer & Manns, 2010; Aggarwal & Naik, 2009).

It has been suggested that the interaction between hepatitis viruses and the innate as well as the adaptive immune system determines the outcome of these infections. Thus, studies regarding specific interactions between viral proteins and components of the immune system may introduce important information about the establishment of chronic infection. Here, we focus on the role of non-parenchymal liver cells and hepatocytes as part of the innate immune system of the liver and their relevance in the pathogenesis of viral hepatitis.

3.1 Hepatitis B virus

Hepatitis B virus is a hepatotropic non-cytopathic DNA virus which belongs to the *Hepadnaviridae* family. An estimated 400 million people worldwide suffer from chronic HBV infection, reaching higher prevalence in Asia and Africa. Patients with chronic infections mostly remain asymptomatic while 10–30% of these individuals develop liver cirrhosis and liver cancer. Although the mechanisms that are involved in viral clearance and persistence are still not fully clarified, it is evident that cell-mediated immune responses play an important role for viral clearance as patients with chronic HBV infection usually fail to develop adequate HBV-specific immune responses. (Bertoletti & Gehring, 2006). Pegylated interferon *a* (IFN-*a*) and nucleos(t)ide analogues are used for therapy of chronic hepatitis B.

3.2 Hepatitis C virus

HCV, a member of the *Flaviviridae family, hepciviridae genius,* is a global health care problem as more than 2% of the world's population (170 million individuals) has been infected with the this hepatotropic virus (Alter, 2007). Infection with HCV leads to chronic hepatitis in 70-80% of the cases, thereby promoting serious hepatic disorders as liver cirrhosis and hepatocellular carcinoma (Di Bisceglie, 1997; Di Bisceglie, 1998). As a consequence, chronic HCV infection is a main indication for liver transplantation. Currently, standard of care is a combination therapy of pegIFN and ribavirin for patients infected with all 6 HCV genotypes (Manns *et al.* 2001), while addition of protease inhibitors have been licensed for the treatment of genotype 1 patients. Recently published clinical trials indicated that triple treatment with the protease inhibitors Telaprevir or Boceprevir in combination with pegIFN and ribavirin, compared to standard treatment with pegIFN and ribavirin alone, significantly improved sustained virologic response rates in naïve patients with HCV genotype 1 infection. In addition, these triple treatments resulted in significantly improved sustained response rates in patients with chronic HCV genotype 1 infection, who were nonresponders or relapsers to previous treatments (Bacon *et al.* 2011; Jacobson *et al.* 2011; Zeuzem *et al.* 2011; Poordad *et al.* 2011).

3.3 Hepatitis D virus

Hepatitis D virus (HDV) has primarily been identified as an additional antigen during HBV infection. It has been shown, that HDV only occurs in HBV infected patients, because it is using HBsAg as envelope protein, which is necessary for the cell entry of HDV (Rizzetto *et al.* 1977; Rizzetto *et al.* 1980). About 20 million HBV infected individuals are thought to be co-infected with HDV, occurring either as a superinfection of chronic HBV infection or a concomitant acute coinfection of HBV and HDV (Hadziyannis, 1997). The pathogenesis of HDV infection is only poorly understood. Whereas clinical observations identified that hepatitis D could be an immune-mediated disease process, specific clinical cases suggested that HDV induces cytopathic infections (Nakano *et al.* 2001). Chronic Hepatitis D is associated with a severe course of hepatitis, frequently leading to rapid fibrosis progression and the development of hepatocellular carcinoma (Wedemeyer & Manns, 2010).

4. Interplay of forces

The local induction of type I IFNs (IFN-α, -β) during the early phase of infection with HBV and HCV (Bigger *et al.* 2001; McClary *et al.* 2000) is crucially important as they are thought to limit HBV as well as HCV replication (Frese *et al.* 2001; Guidotti *et al.* 1994) while induction of IFN-γ during progression of viral infection may additionally inhibit viral replication (Frese *et al.* 2002; Guidotti *et al.* 1996).

4.1 Innate immunity against HBV

The role of the innate immune system during the early phase of HBV infection has been investigated in different experimental systems. Wieland *et al.* investigated the transcriptome of the liver in three chimpanzees during the course of acute HBV infection (Wieland *et al.* 2004). Their analysis focused on two diverse groups of cellular genes: those in the early phase are associated with the innate immune response, and those in the late phase are associated with the adaptive immune response that terminates infection. They demonstrated that this virus does not induce any genes during entry and expansion, leading the authors to suggest that HBV is a 'stealth virus' in the early phase of infection. By contrast, a large number of IFN-γ-regulated genes are expressed in the liver during viral clearance (Figure 3). This upregulation of IFN-γ-regulated genes in livers results from the adaptive T cell response as specific T-cells infiltrating the liver are major producers of IFN-γ (Wieland *et al.* 2004). Thus, HBV and HCV infections strongly differ in the early phase of infection, as HCV induces a strong IFN-α response in chimpanzees (Su *et al.* 2002).

There are data to suggest that HBV actively inhibits the induction of an early IFN response. Wu *et al.* showed a regulatory effect of TLR-activated KC and LSEC on the *in vitro* replication of HBV in a co-culture model utilizing HBV-Met cells (Pasquetto *et al.* 2002). TLR3- and TLR4-activated KC as well as TLR3-activated LSEC induced a MyD88-independent response inhibiting HBV replication. While HBV replicative intermediates were highly suppressed, viral mRNAs as well as secretion of HBsAg and HBeAg remained largely unchanged. The HBV suppressing effect mediated by TLR3 ligands was caused by IFN-β whereas TLR4-activated KC additionally induced undefined cytokines with antiviral activity (Wu *et al.* 2007).

Further studies included co-culture experiments with hepatocytes or NPC and HBV-Met cell supernatants, HBsAg, HBeAg as well as HBV virions resulting in abrogation of TLR-induced antiviral activity, correlating with decreased activation of IRF-3, NFκB and ERK1/2. In comparison to primary hepatocytes, HBV-infected HBV-Met cells did not induce antiviral cytokines upon TLR activation. TLR-induced expression of TNF-α and IL-6 was suppressed in the presence of high amounts of HBV. Accordingly, suppression of HBV replication by siRNA leads to activation or expression of pro-inflammatory transcription factors and cytokines (Wu *et al.* 2008). These data might explain why HBV does not induce a strong initial type I IFN response such as HCV and, therefore, behaves as a 'stealth virus' (Wieland *et al.* 2004).

Despite of the fact that HBV does not induce an IFN response during the early phase of infection, it can be recognized by liver resident cells, thereby activating innate immune responses without IFN induction. Hoesel *et al.* recently showed that HBV is recognized by hepatic NPC, mainly by Kupffer cells, upon infection of primary human liver cells *in vitro*. Within 3 hours, these cells release inflammatory cytokines including IL-1β, -6, -8 and TNF-α without inducing an IFN response. NFκB-dependent IL-6 secretion of activated KC is able to control HBV gene expression and replication in hepatocytes at the level of transcription. IL-6 leads to activation of MAPKs exogenous signal-regulated kinase (ERK) 1/2 and c-jun N-terminal kinase resulting in decreased expression of two transcription factors (hepatocyte nuclear factor (HNF) 1α and HNF 4α) that are essential for HBV gene expression and replication (Hoesel *et al.* 2009).

A recent publication studied the full replication cycle of hepatitis B virus (HBV) in primary hepatocyte cultures that were isolated from the northern treeshrew (*Tupaia belangeri*). The Tupaia model has been used to investigate the effect of cytokines on HBV infection. Stimulation of HBV infected primary Tupaia hepatocytes with recombinant Tupaia TNF-α led to viral suppression while covalently closed circular DNA and viral RNA were still detectable leading to the conclusion that TNF-α may also control HBV infection (Xu *et al.* 2011).

Consistently, Zhang *et al.* demonstrated that activation of cellular pathways by TLR ligands leads to inhibition of hepadnaviral replication (Zhang *et al.* 2009). Using the model of woodchuck hepatitis virus (WHV) infected primary hepatocytes (PWH), Poly I:C and LPS stimulation resulted in upregulation of cellular antiviral genes and TLRs. LPS stimulation led to a pronounced reduction of WHV replication intermediates without a significant IFN induction while Poly I:C transfection resulted in the production of IFN and a highly increased expression of antiviral genes in PWHs and slight inhibitory effect on WHV replication. LPS could activate NFκB, MAPK, and PI-3k/Akt pathways in PWHs. Furthermore, inhibitors of MAPK-ERK and PI-3k/Akt pathways, but not those of IFN signaling pathways, were able to block the antiviral effect of LPS. These results indicate that IFN-independent pathways which activated by LPS are able to down-regulate hepadnaviral replication in hepatocytes (Zhang *et al.* 2009).

A direct activation of cellular pathways through the expression of cellular adaptors involved in signaling has similar effects like the stimulation with TLR ligands. Guo *et al.* determined the effects of PRR-mediated innate immune response on HBV replication in hepatoma cell lines. Plasmids expressing TLR adaptors, MyD88, TRIF, or RIG-I/MDA5 adaptor or interferon promoter stimulator 1 (IPS-1) were transfected into cells and led to dramatic reduction of the levels of HBV mRNA and DNA in hepatoma cells. Analysis of involved signaling pathways revealed that activation of NFκB is required for all three adaptors to elicit antiviral response in both HepG2 and Huh7 cells while activation of IRF-3 is only essential for induction of antiviral response by IPS-1 in Huh7 cells (Guo *et al.* 2009).

Although recent publications consistently confirmed the antiviral role of TLR-mediated innate responses of hepatic cells, the antiviral mechanisms that are induced by activation of the TLR system are not fully understood. IFN-β has been identified as the major antiviral factor produced by NPCs in response to TLR3 and 4 ligands (Wu *et al.* 2007). Wieland *et al.* showed that IFN-β inhibits hepatitis B virus (HBV) replication by non-cytolytic mechanisms that either destabilize pregenomic (pg)RNA-containing capsids or prevent their assembly. Using a doxycycline (dox)-inducible HBV replication system, IFN-β pretreatment led to production of replication-competent pgRNA-containing capsids. The turnover rate of preformed HBV RNA-containing capsids is not changed in the presence of IFN-β or IFN-γ.

These conditions further inhibited pgRNA synthesis. Thus, type I and II IFNs prevent the formation of replication-competent HBV capsids (Wieland *et al.* 2005). IL-6 was shown to activate cellular signaling pathways in PHHs including the MAPK pathway and inhibit the HBV gene transcription (Hoesel *et al.* 2009). In PWHs infected with WHV, LPS activates the MAPK pathway and reduce the WHV replication, but unable to deplete WHV transcripts (Zhang *et al.* 2009). Future studies are necessary to clarify the mechanisms involved in TLR-mediated anti-HBV actions.

As TLR-mediated immune responses down regulate HBV replication, HBV developed mechanisms to counteract these antiviral functions. Hepatocytes and Kupffer cells isolated from liver biopsies of patients with chronic hepatitis B (CHB) showed significantly decreased expression of TLR2 on hepatocytes, KCs and peripheral monocytes in patients with HBeAg-positive CHB in comparison with HBeAg negative CHB and controls (steatosis patients). The level of TLR4 expression did not significantly differ between these groups. Hepatic cell lines harboring a recombinant baculovirus encoding HBV significantly reduced TNF-α expression as well as phospho-p38 kinase expression in the presence of HBeAg. Within the absence of HBeAg, HBV replication was associated with upregulation of the TLR2 pathway resulting in increased TNF-α expression (Visvanathan *et al.* 2007). Consistent with these findings, the TLR expression was significantly suppressed in liver tissue and PBMC of woodchucks chronically infected with WHV, assuming an important role of TLR2 during hepadnaviral infection and pathogenesis (Zhang *et al.* unpublished). HBV additionally blocked the gene expression of MyD88, an essential adaptor molecule in TLR-mediated innate immune responses. The terminal protein (TP) domain of the HBV polymerase was described to be responsible for this antagonistic activity. It is supposed that the HBV polymerase inhibits IFN-inducible MyD88 expression by blocking the nuclear translocation of STAT1 and therefore representing a general inhibitor of IFN signaling (Wu *et al.* 2007).

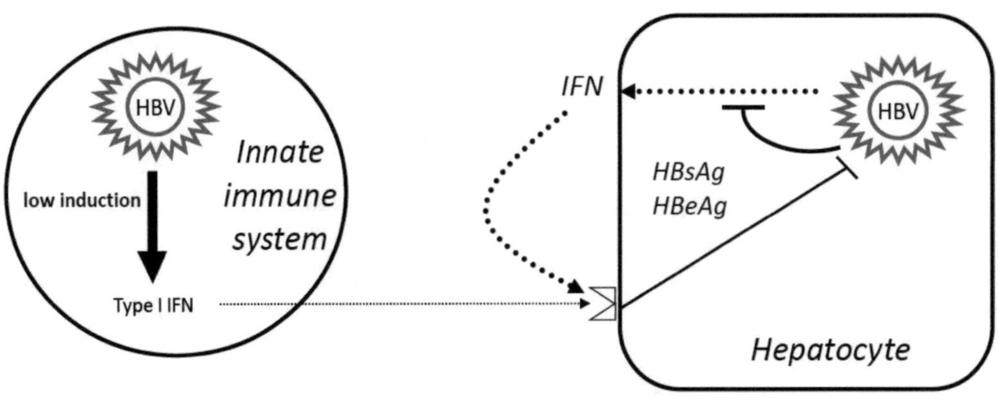

Fig. 3. Role of the innate immunity during pathogenesis of HBV
HBV infection only induces a weak type I IFN response. HBsAg or HBeAg inhibit endogenous expression of IFNs in the early phase of infection .Activated cells of the innate immune system may still produce type I IFNs , therefore limiting viral replication.

Isogawa *et al.* examined the ability of different TLRs to effect HBV replication *in vivo*. HBV transgenic mice have been injected with single doses of TLR2, -3, -4, -5, -7 and -9 ligands.

With the exception for TLR2, all of the ligands suppressed HBV replication in the liver in an IFN-α/-β-dependent manner (Isogawa *et al.* 2005). The potential of these TLR ligands to provoke the expression of antiviral cytokines at the site of HBV replication, leads to suggestion that TLR activation represents a powerful tool for novel therapeutic strategies in the treatment of chronic HBV infection.

4.2 Innate immunity against HCV

Standard treatment of HCV infection is the combination of pegylated type I IFN and ribavirin. Interferons are antiviral cytokines, produced after activation of the innate immune system during virus infection. Secretion of IFN leads neighbouring cells to switch to an 'antiviral state' and resists viral infection. Thus, an important role of the innate immune system is to limit viral replication and spread as well as to promote and orchestrate subsequent adaptive immune reactions. While the mechanisms that are utilized by the innate immune system to control HCV infection are not well defined, it is generally accepted that IFN signaling is likely to be involved. Viral proteins are able to potently activate the innate immune system. Nevertheless, HCV developed different mechanisms to evolve cellular, antiviral and innate immune responses, reflecting the adaptation to its host.
Molecular patterns within the 5' as well as the 3' non-translated region (NTR) of the HCV genome have been identified as retinoic acid inducible gene I (RIG-I) activating PAMPs. RIG-I is a well characterized PRR sensing and affecting HCV replication. Binding of viral double stranded RNA to the cytosolic RNA helicase RIG-I recruits the mitochondria-associated CARDIF protein, which induces IKKε/TBK1 kinases-mediated IRF-3 phosphorylation and thereby induces IFN-β expression. It is supposed that HCV RNA initiates IFN-β secretion in a RIG-I-dependent manner through its 5' and 3' NTR secondary structure (Saito *et al.* 2007; McCormick *et al.* 2004; Sumpter, Jr. *et al.* 2005). It has been additionally demonstrated that TLR3 is able to detect HCV structures in cultured hepatoma cells, leading to activation of IRF-3 and expression of ISGs, which limit HCV replication. The HCV motif that triggers TLR3 signaling remains to be characterized (Wang *et al.* 2009). It is suggested that RIG-I and TLR3 represent independent signaling pathways that are involved in IRF-3- and NFκB-mediated antiviral state during HCV infection (Alexopoulou *et al.* 2001; Yoneyama *et al.* 2004) (Figure 4).
In defiance of this immune activation HCV is able to subvert the antiviral activity of the innate immune system. Recent data suggested that the viral NS3/4A serine protease of the Hepatitis C virus may enable its persistent infection. The NS3/4A protein causes specific proteolysis of the TRIF adaptor molecule downstream the TLR3 signaling. It has been demonstrated that the viral NS3/4A protease additionally leads to disruption of RIG-I signaling. Therefore the viral NS3/4A protease cleaves CARDIF and abrogates IKKε/TBK1-mediated IFN-β secretion (Li *et al.* 2005; Foy *et al.* 2005; Foy *et al.* 2003; Breiman *et al.* 2005; Vilasco *et al.* 2006).
Broering *et al.* and Wang *et al.* investigated the antiviral capacity of TLR-activated KC, LSEC and HSC against HCV. Despite the expression of all TLRs, murine KC and LSEC only suppressed HCV replication in a co-culture model after activation of TLR3 and -4 which were mediated by IFN-β only (Broering *et al.* 2008). Similar results were obtained for murine HSC. Here, IFN-β was responsible for the antiviral activity of TLR3-stimulated HSC, whereas additional cytokines of undefined nature seem to be involved in the TLR4-mediated antiviral effect. In case of human HSC, only TLR3 stimulation led to production of

antiviral cytokines. HCV suppression was related to the upregulation of ISGs and RIG-I in target cells (Wang *et al.* 2009).

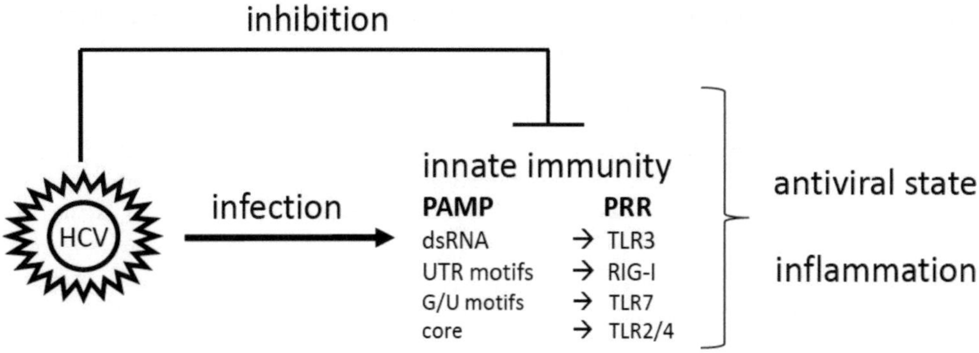

Fig. 4. HCV triggers innate immunity
Different structures of the hepatitis C virus can be detected by the innate immune system. This leads to cytokine secretion and induction of an antiviral state as well as inflammation processes. The virus developed evading strategies to subvert this antiviral state.

Recently established HCV cell culture models (Lindenbach *et al.* 2005; Wakita *et al.* 2005; Zhong *et al.* 2005) lead to the generation of infectious HCV particles. Zhang *et al.* generated cell culture derived HCV particles to study their immunomodulatory effects on freshly isolated PBMCs and pDCs obtained from healthy blood donors. While complete HCV particles were not able to induce cytokine production, purified HCV RNA led to immune stimulation, accompanied by enhanced TLR7 activation. It was suggested that the HCV RNA genome contains G/U-rich motifs which have immune-stimulatory capacity. It is hypothesized that HCV particles are digested by endosomal proteases, the uncoated viral genomes and therefore the G/U-rich motifs mediate TLR7 activation (Diebold *et al.* 2004; Jurk *et al.* 2002). Lee *et al.* additionally revealed an interaction between TLR7 and HCV, wherein TLR7 mediates interferon secretion as well as interferon-independent immune responses (Lee *et al.* 2006). Further analysis indicated a higher prevalence of single nucleotide polymorphisms (SNP) in TLR7 of patients chronically infected with HCV. These SNPs significantly correlates with the progression of liver fibrosis in patients with chronic HCV infection (Schott *et al.* 2007).

Another mechanism of HCV to evade the attack of the innate immune system targets TLR7. A significant decrease in TLR7 expression was shown in the presence of HCV *in vitro* and *in vivo* (Chang *et al.* 2010). It was proposed that HCV directly interferes with the transcriptional regulation of TLR7 mRNA. HCV replication level directly correlates with TLR7 expression, as reconstitution of TLR7 expression levels were achieved upon viral suppression. Despite this decrease in TLR7 mRNA in HCV-replicating cells, increased activation of IRF-7 was detected. This indicates that other PRR induce nuclear translocation of IRF-7 in HCV replicating cells (Chang *et al.* 2010).

Innate immunity is additionally activated by the HCV core protein leading to inflammation but failing to induce antiviral cytokines (Dolganiuc *et al.* 2004; Feldmann *et al.* 2006). Other studies have described that synthetic lipopeptide-complexes of the HCV core protein mediate the innate immune response through TLR2 and TLR4 (Duesberg *et al.* 2002). In

addition, an increased expression of some TLRs as well as inflammatory cytokines was shown in PBMC of chronically infected HCV patients (Sato *et al.* 2007).
Dolganiuc *et al.* identified pre-activated monocytes in patients with chronic hepatitis C. In this study, increased IFN-γ, endotoxin and HCV core protein seemed to modulate monocyte functions, resulting in the generation of MyD88/IRAK complexes, NFκB activation and increased expression of TNF-α. These findings lead the authors to suggest that LPS, HCV core protein and IFN-γ extend the activation of inflammatory monocytes/macrophages indicating a loss of TLR tolerance. These observations additionally lead to the assumption, that both host- as well as virus-derived factors influence macrophages to mediate persistent inflammation during chronic HCV infection (Dolganiuc *et al.* 2007).

4.2.1 Interferon response; friend or foe?

Elevated hepatic ISG expression in HCV infected chimpanzees as well as in patients was identified as a virus induced type I IFN response (Bigger *et al.* 2001; Bigger *et al.* 2004; Helbig *et al.* 2005). As already discussed HCV developed evading strategies to subvert the innate immune system. While infected cells are not able to sense the virus and subsequently secrete IFNs, it is supposed that the increased ISG expression during HCV infection is induced by an activated local innate immune system. Activation of the innate immune system, NPCs in particular, results in the expression and secretion of IFN-β. Type I IFNs bind to their cell surface receptor leading to conformational changes, which activate the Janus kinase - Signal Transducers and Activators of Transcription (JAK–STAT) signaling pathways. Downstream phosphorylation of STAT-1 and STAT-2 recruits a third factor (IRF-9) forming the transcription-complex ISG factor-3 (ISGF-3). ISGF-3 translocates into the nucleus and interacts with IFN stimulated response elements (ISRE) in the promoter regions of ISGs. Expression of selected ISGs may result in HCV eradication in acute hepatitis C infection (Bigger *et al.* 2001). However, progression of persistent HCV infection can be established due to escape strategies against the immune system which may also be responsible for non-response to therapies that are based upon the administration of exogenous IFNs (Sato *et al.* 2007).
A subgroup of ISGs has been described to directly suppress HCV replication. Protein kinase R (PKR) for example, phosphorylates the alpha subunit of the eukaryotic initiation factor (eIF)-2 leading to suppression of translational processes (Gale, Jr. *et al.* 1999; Pflugheber *et al.* 2002). The RNA-specific adenosine deaminase 1 (ADAR1) binds to dsRNA resulting in destabilization of secondary structures (Taylor *et al.* 2005). The antiviral function of 2′-5′ oligoadenylate synthetases (2′-5′ OAS) is mediated by the activation of the latently expressed endoribonuclease RNaseL, which induce degradation of viral and cellular RNA (Silverman, 1994; Zhou *et al.* 1997). ISG56 is an IRF-3 responsive gene that blocks one of the eIF3 subunits resulting in inhibition of translation (Wang *et al.* 2003; Hui *et al.* 2003; Terenzi *et al.* 2005). Additional ISGs affecting HCV replication have been identified during IFN therapy including MxA, ISG 6–16 and Viperin. The mechanisms of action of these host factors are still unclear (Bigger *et al.* 2004; Helbig *et al.* 2005; Suzuki *et al.* 2004).
HCV evolved mechanisms to influence this type I IFN response induced by the JAK–STAT signaling. The HCV polyprotein has been described as a strong inhibitor of IFN-α-induced signaling, as it impairs ISGF3 DNA binding. This effect is mediated by an increase in STAT1–protein inhibitor of activated STAT1 (PIAS1) association, resulting in the decreased transcriptional activity of ISGF3 through hypomethylation of STAT1 (Blindenbacher *et al.*

2003; Heim *et al.* 1999). In addition, also HCV core protein effects JAK-STAT signaling. The core protein induces STAT1 degradation, inhibits STAT1 activation/phosphorylation and increases the induction of suppressor of cytokine signaling (SOCS) proteins (Bode *et al.* 2003; Lin *et al.* 2005; Lin *et al.* 2006). Furthermore, the core protein suppresses the binding capacity of ISGF3 to the ISRE, resulting in decreased expression of anti-HCV effective ISG (de Lucas *et al.* 2005). Moreover, HCV proteins directly inhibit the antiviral action of selected ISGs. The envelope protein E2 and the non-structural protein NS5A have been reported as antagonists of PKR, leading to the disruption of translation control by IFNs (Gale, Jr. *et al.* 1998; Taylor *et al.* 1999).

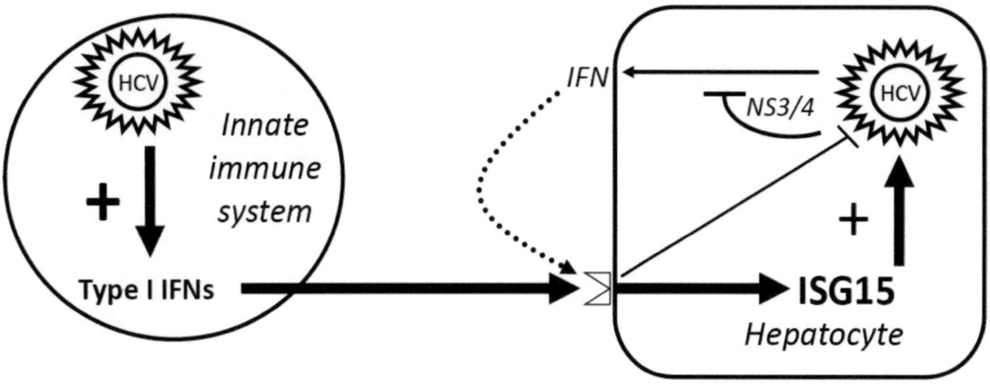

Fig. 5. Role of the innate immunity in the pathogenesis of HCV infection
HCV may directly induce type IFNs, while viral proteins like NS3/4 can inhibit endogenous expression of IFNs. Activated cells of the innate immune system might still produce type I IFNs resulting in increased ISG15 expression in infected cells and therefore promoting HCV replication.

The local type I IFN response induced by HCV seems to be paradox, as these interferons can inhibit HCV replication. In addition, patients that are non-responders to IFN-based therapies have highly elevated expression levels of a subset of ISGs compared to patients who cleared the virus (Asselah *et al.* 2008; Chen *et al.* 2005). ISG15, an ubiquitin-like modifier, is one of these genes. ISG15 is conjugated to a subset of target proteins. The functional consequence of this ISGylation is still unclear. ISGylated proteins are not degraded by the proteasome as ubiquitinylated proteins are (Malakhov *et al.* 2002; Ritchie & Zhang, 2004). Recently published data indicate that ISGylation negatively modulates interferon signaling (Chua *et al.* 2009; Broering *et al.* 2010), in addition ISGylation and ISG15 itself directly promote HCV replication (Chen *et al.* 2010; Broering *et al.* 2010). These observations may explain why elevated expression of ISGs, and ISG15 in particular, during HCV infection is beneficial for the hepatitis C virus (Figure 5).

4.3 Innate immunity against HDV

There are only few studies on the interaction of HDV with host innate responses. Like many other viruses, HDV seems to have developed anti-IFN-α strategies as it negatively affects the activation of IFN-α signaling by interfering the JAK-STAT signal transduction pathway. An early publication from McNair *et al.* demonstrated that neither IFN-α nor IFN-γ was able to inhibit HDV gene expression and formation of genomic and antigenomic RNA in cell lines stably transfected HDV genomes (McNair *et al.* 1994). However, such cell lines showed no defect in upregulation of ISGs like PKR, 2′-5′ OAS and IRF-1 or in induction of an antiviral status after IFN treatment. These cells were able to upregulate IFN-β after Poly I:C treatment. The presence of HDV RNA did not affect PKR function.

In contrast, Pugnale *et al.* showed in a transient tranfection system that hepatoma cells replicating HDV have an impaired response to IFN-α (Pugnale *et al.* 2009). By unknown mechanisms, the phosphorylation of both STAT-1 and STAT-2 was greatly impaired, consequently, both factors did not relocate into the nucleus. In addition, the IFN-α stimulated tyrosine phosphorylation of IFN receptor-associated JAK kinase Tyk2 was also inhibited by HDV, without affecting either the tyrosine phosphorylation of Jak1 or the expression of type I IFN receptor subunits. Both studies showed consistently that IFNs are not able to suppress HDV. Pugnale *et al.* could detect the inhibition of IFN signaling in HDV replicating cells, likely due to the higher levels of viral RNA and proteins in the transient transfection system (Pugnale *et al.* 2009). Despite of the dsRNA nature of HDV genomic and antigenomic RNAs, there was no apparent activation of IFN pathways in the stably transfected cell lines, indicating that HDV RNA may be sequestered during replication (McNair *et al.* 1994).

Another report demonstrated that large HDV antigen (L-HDAg) may enhance the ISG MxA more than 3-fold. However, the upregulation of MxA by IFN-α is generally very strong and may reach levels of more than 100-fold compared to unstimulated controls. Thus, the ability of L-HDAg to activate ISG expression is rather low (Williams *et al.* 2009). Thus, HDV is a weak inducer of cellular IFN responses and is likely able to inhibit IFN signaling. In addition, it has also been reported that IFN-α inducible protein ADAR1 modulates HDV gene expression and genome replication by editing the HDV genome (Hartwig *et al.* 2004).

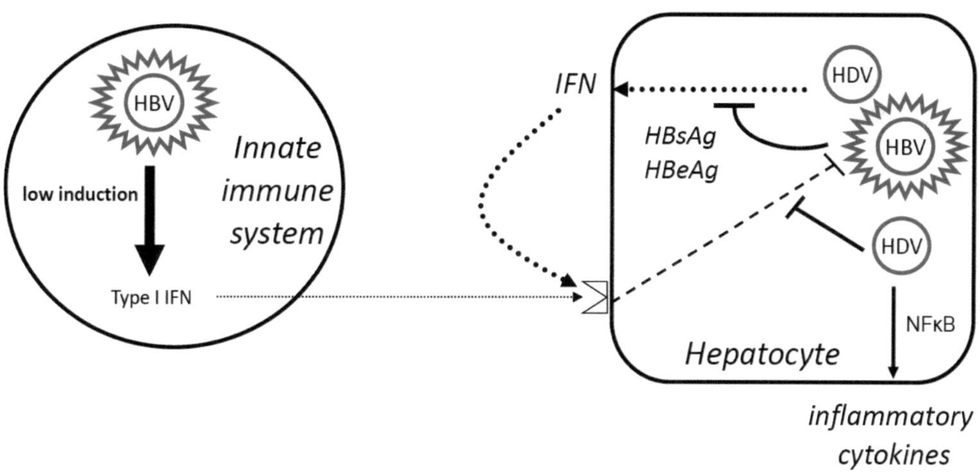

Fig. 6. Role of the innate immunity during pathogenesis of HBV HDV coinfection
HBV as well as HDV only induce a weak type IFN response. HBsAg or HBeAg are supposed to inhibit endogenous expression of IFNs. Activated cells of the innate immune system might still produce type I IFNs. HDV is able to block JAK/STAT signaling, thereby subverting the IFN response. HDV additionally promotes NFκB activation and secretion of inflammatory cytokines.

NFκB activation is involved in many inflammatory processes and in cancer. The L-HDAg has been shown to mediate TNF-α-induced NFκB signaling, probably through the direct association with TRAF2, a protein implicating the early signaling events (Park *et al.* 2009). Several studies revealed a relationship between L-HDAg, S-HDAg, genomic RNA or antigenomic RNA and the proteome of the cell (Mota *et al.* 2009; Mota *et al.* 2008). Modified expression profile of proteins involving regulation of nucleic acid and protein metabolism, energy pathways, signal transduction, transport, apoptosis and cell growth were found. Host factors involved in HDV replication have been determind using a small inhibitory RNA (siRNA) screening. Cells stably trasfected with the S-HDAg were treated with siRNA before HDV infection (Cao *et al.* 2009). It has been reported that a part of the genome, described as an RNA promoter, directy interacts with some cellular proteins (Beard *et al.* 1996) (Figure 6).

It could be demonstrated that two of these host factors, the eukaryotic translation elongation factor 1 alpha 1 (eEF1A1) and the glyceraldehyde-3-phosphate dehydrogenase (GAPDH), are involved in RNA processing and in the translation machinery. Of note, these genes are often considered and used as housekeeping genes (Sikora *et al.* 2009).

5. Coinfection of HBV and HCV

Clinical investigations on disease outcomes and progression in patients coinfected with HBV and HCV are diverse and contradictory. Viral interference or reciprocal replicative suppression of the two viruses probably occurs (Liaw *et al.* 1994; Zarski *et al.* 1998). Due to a missing model system for HBV/HCV coinfection in the past, virological and molecular aspects are poorly understood (Brass & Moradpour, 2009). Resent studies investigated the mechanisms of HBV and HCV coinfection by heterologous overexpression of viral proteins, leading to conflicting results. It has been demonstrated that the HCV core protein and NS5A negatively regulate HBV replication, whereas other studies could not confirm these findings (Pasquinelli *et al.* 1997; Chen *et al.* 2003; Schuttler *et al.* 2002).

It seems to be important to address the question whether direct interference occurs between the viruses in order to understand the disease progression. Recent studies have addressed this issue (Eyre *et al.* 2009; Bellecave *et al.* 2009). The human hepatoma cell line Huh-7 supports HBV replication and formation of HBV virions. Huh-7 cells also can be used to study the HCV life cycle, including viral entry, RNA replication and release of infectious particles. Using this cell culture system, these authors independently showed that HBV and HCV are able to replicate in the same cell, without showing interfering processes. HBV replicating cells can be infected with cell culture-derived HCV resulting in secretion of infectious HCV. In addition, the inhibition of one of these viruses did not influence the replication of the other. It is well known that HBV replication, for example, may be suppressed in the presence of replicative HCV infection while eradication of HCV may lead to replicative activity of HBV infection. This phenomenon may be explained by the fact that HCV may induce local IFN production by NPCs through activation of TLR3 which may lead to suppression of HBV replication (Broering *et al.* 2008; Wu *et al.* 2007) (Figure 7).

6. Conclusions

TLRs have been identified as key regulators of innate and adaptive immune responses in the liver as they play a critical role in the pathogenesis and progression of many liver diseases as well as in the regulation of tissue injury and wound healing processes. The local innate immune system represented by hepatocytes, liver sinusoidal endothelial cells, Kupffer cells and stellate cells, for example, is involved in the induction of systemic tolerance or inflammation and additionally cross-talks to the adaptive immune system. It has been suggested that the local innate immune system is of importance in the progression of HBV or HCV infection. PRRs, especially TLRs play a pivotal role in the pathogenesis of viral hepatitis due to their rapid signal transduction. It has been clearly demonstrated that TLRs participate in antiviral immunity.

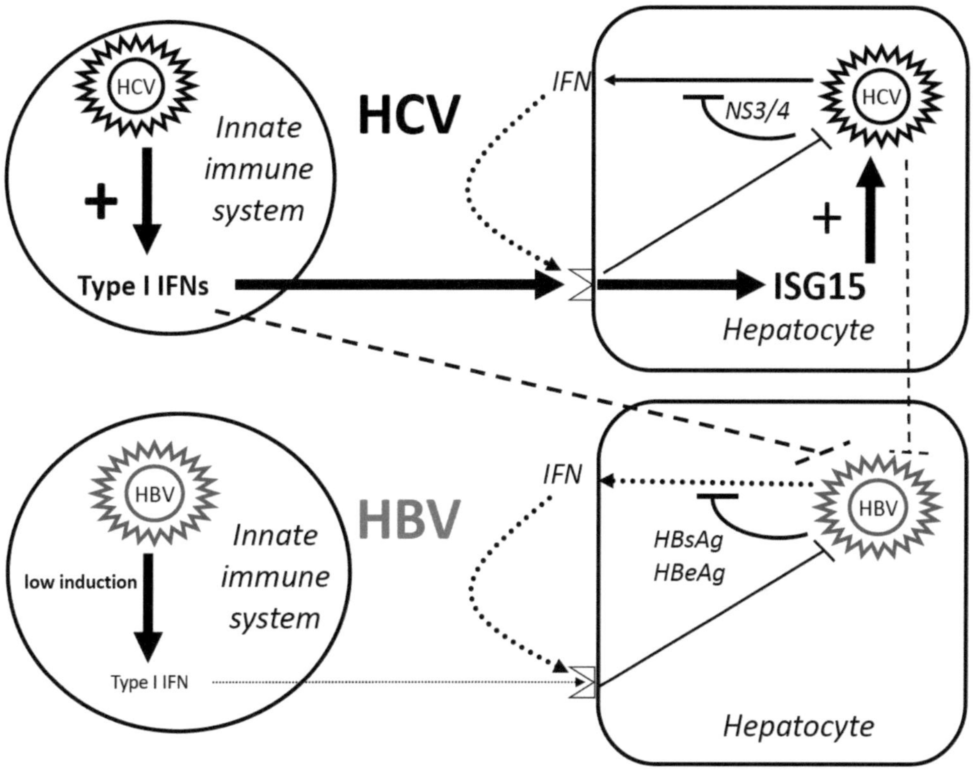

Fig. 7. Role of the innate immunity during pathogenesis of viral hepatitis
HCV infection directly induces type IFNs, later viral proteins like NS3/4 inhibits endogenous expression of IFNs. Activated cells of the innate immune system might still produce type I IFNs resulting in increased ISG15 expression in infected cells and therefore promoting HCV replication. HBV likewise seems to inhibit endogenous IFN expression, additionally inhibiting TLR activation in the local immune system. This may explain way HCV but not HBV induce an initial type I IFN response during acute infection. In case of HBV/HCV co-infection, HCV-activated NPC may inhibit HBV replication by the production of type I IFNs.

As a consequence, various evading strategies have been evolved by hepatitis viruses (HBV, HCV and HDV) to counteract these antiviral activities:
The hepatic innate immune system is able to sense PAMP structures of these hepatotropic viruses, resulting in secretion of antiviral cytokines, in particular interferons, and therefore

limits viral replication. Conversely, the hepatitis viruses may counteract and subvert the innate immunity by evolutionary adaptation.
The Hepatitis B virus for example developed a mechanism to block the expression of interferon sensitive genes, especially MyD88, an adaptor molecule involved in mostly all of the TLR signaling parthways. In addition HBV evades the TLR2 signaling, which results in limitation of viral replication, by directly decreasing its expression. These evasion strategies may explain the absence of an antiviral response during infection and the description as a 'stealth virus'. Coinfection with Hepatitis D virus is additionally accompanied by further evasion of the IFN response.
In contrast to this Hepatitis C virus initially induces a strong type I IFN response. However, the virus is able to control this antiviral signaling by evasion strategies directly targeting the TLR3 or RIG-I pathway, which initiate IFN-β expression. In addition, HCV developed different mechanisms to block the JAK-STAT signaling, resulting in abrogation of the IFN response, in particular the expression of ISGs with antiviral functions. HCV paradoxically needs one of these response genes, ISG15, which promotes HCV replication and negatively regulates the IFN response.
These evolutionary developed adaptations of HBC, HCV and HDV to their host invert the benefits of the antiviral response, induced by the local innate immune system. The inadequate but consistent activation of the hepatic innate immunity results in tolerance induction and permits progression of viral persistence and chronic infections. Therefore, therapeutic manipulations of the hepatic TLR pathways are of high interest for the development of novel treatment strategies.

7. References

Aggarwal, R., Naik, S. 2009, Epidemiology of hepatitis E: current status, J. Gastroenterol. Hepatol., 24(9), pp. 1484-1493.

Akira, S., Takeda, K. 2004, Toll-like receptor signalling, Nat.Rev.Immunol., 4(7), pp. 499-511.

Akira, S., Uematsu, S., Takeuchi, O. 2006, Pathogen recognition and innate immunity, Cell, 124(4), pp. 783-801.

Alexopoulou, L., Holt, A. C., Medzhitov, R., Flavell, R. A. 2001, Recognition of double-stranded RNA and activation of NF-kappaB by Toll-like receptor 3, Nature, 413(6857), pp. 732-738.

Alter, M. J. 2007, Epidemiology of hepatitis C virus infection, World J.Gastroenterol., 13(17), pp. 2436-2441.

Asselah, T., Bieche, I., Narguet, S., Sabbagh, A., Laurendeau, I., Ripault, M. P., Boyer, N., Martinot-Peignoux, M., Valla, D., Vidaud, M., Marcellin, P. 2008, Liver gene expression signature to predict response to pegylated interferon plus ribavirin combination therapy in patients with chronic hepatitis C, Gut, 57(4), pp. 516-524.

Bacon, B. R., Gordon, S. C., Lawitz, E., Marcellin, P., Vierling, J. M., Zeuzem, S., Poordad, F., Goodman, Z. D., Sings, H. L., Boparai, N., Burroughs, M., Brass, C. A., Albrecht, J. K., Esteban, R. 2011, Boceprevir for previously treated chronic HCV genotype 1 infection, N.Engl.J.Med., 364(13), pp. 1207-1217.

Beard, M. R., MacNaughton, T. B., Gowans, E. J. 1996, Identification and characterization of a hepatitis delta virus RNA transcriptional promoter, J.Virol., 70(8), pp. 4986-4995.

Bellecave, P., Gouttenoire, J., Gajer, M., Brass, V., Koutsoudakis, G., Blum, H. E., Bartenschlager, R., Nassal, M., Moradpour, D. 2009, Hepatitis B and C virus coinfection: a novel model system reveals the absence of direct viral interference, Hepatology, 50(1), pp. 46-55.

Bertoletti, A., Gehring, A. J. 2006, The immune response during hepatitis B virus infection, J.Gen.Virol., 87(Pt 6), pp. 1439-1449.

Bigger, C. B., Brasky, K. M., Lanford, R. E. 2001, DNA microarray analysis of chimpanzee liver during acute resolving hepatitis C virus infection, J.Virol., 75(15), pp. 7059-7066.

Bigger, C. B., Guerra, B., Brasky, K. M., Hubbard, G., Beard, M. R., Luxon, B. A., Lemon, S. M., Lanford, R. E. 2004, Intrahepatic gene expression during chronic hepatitis C virus infection in chimpanzees, J.Virol., 78(24), pp. 13779-13792.

Biron, C. A. 1998, Role of early cytokines, including alpha and beta interferons (IFN-alpha/beta), in innate and adaptive immune responses to viral infections, Semin.Immunol., 10(5), pp. 383-390.

Blindenbacher, A., Duong, F. H., Hunziker, L., Stutvoet, S. T., Wang, X., Terracciano, L., Moradpour, D., Blum, H. E., Alonzi, T., Tripodi, M., La, M. N., Heim, M. H. 2003, Expression of hepatitis c virus proteins inhibits interferon alpha signaling in the liver of transgenic mice, Gastroenterology, 124(5), pp. 1465-1475.

Bode, J. G., Ludwig, S., Ehrhardt, C., Albrecht, U., Erhardt, A., Schaper, F., Heinrich, P. C., Haussinger, D. 2003, IFN-alpha antagonistic activity of HCV core protein involves induction of suppressor of cytokine signaling-3, FASEB J., 17(3), pp. 488-490.

Brass, V., Moradpour, D. 2009, New insights into hepatitis B and C virus co-infection, J.Hepatol., 51(3), pp. 423-425.

Breiman, A., Grandvaux, N., Lin, R., Ottone, C., Akira, S., Yoneyama, M., Fujita, T., Hiscott, J., Meurs, E. F. 2005, Inhibition of RIG-I-dependent signaling to the interferon pathway during hepatitis C virus expression and restoration of signaling by IKKepsilon, J.Virol., 79(7), pp. 3969-3978.

Broering, R., Wu, J., Meng, Z., Hilgard, P., Lu, M., Trippler, M., Szczeponek, A., Gerken, G., Schlaak, J. F. 2008, Toll-like receptor-stimulated non-parenchymal liver cells can regulate hepatitis C virus replication, J.Hepatol., 48(6), pp. 914-922.

Broering, R., Zhang, X., Kottilil, S., Trippler, M., Jiang, M., Lu, M., Gerken, G., Schlaak, J. F. 2010, The interferon stimulated gene 15 functions as a proviral factor for the hepatitis C virus and as a regulator of the IFN response, Gut, 59(8), pp. 1111-1119.

Cao, D., Haussecker, D., Huang, Y., Kay, M. A. 2009, Combined proteomic-RNAi screen for host factors involved in human hepatitis delta virus replication, RNA., 15(11), pp. 1971-1979.

Chang, S., Kodys, K., Szabo, G. 2010a, Impaired expression and function of toll-like receptor 7 in hepatitis C virus infection in human hepatoma cells, Hepatology, 51(1), pp. 35-42.

Chen, L., Borozan, I., Feld, J., Sun, J., Tannis, L. L., Coltescu, C., Heathcote, J., Edwards, A. M., McGilvray, I. D. 2005, Hepatic gene expression discriminates responders and nonresponders in treatment of chronic hepatitis C viral infection, Gastroenterology, 128(5), pp. 1437-1444.

Chen, L., Sun, J., Meng, L., Heathcote, J., Edwards, A. M., McGilvray, I. D. 2010, ISG15, a ubiquitin-like interferon-stimulated gene, promotes hepatitis C virus production in vitro: implications for chronic infection and response to treatment, J.Gen.Virol., 91(Pt 2), pp. 382-388.

Chen, S. Y., Kao, C. F., Chen, C. M., Shih, C. M., Hsu, M. J., Chao, C. H., Wang, S. H., You, L. R., Lee, Y. H. 2003, Mechanisms for inhibition of hepatitis B virus gene expression and replication by hepatitis C virus core protein, J.Biol.Chem., 278(1), pp. 591-607.

Chua, P. K., McCown, M. F., Rajyaguru, S., Kular, S., Varma, R., Symons, J., Chiu, S. S., Cammack, N., Najera, I. 2009, Modulation of the Interferon {alpha} Anti-Hepatitis C Virus Activity by ISG15, J.Gen.Virol..

de Lucas S., Bartolome, J., Carreno, V. 2005, Hepatitis C virus core protein down-regulates transcription of interferon-induced antiviral genes, J.Infect.Dis., 191(1), pp. 93-99.

Di Bisceglie, A. M. 1997, Hepatitis C and hepatocellular carcinoma, Hepatology, 26(3 Suppl 1), pp. 34S-38S.

Di Bisceglie, A. M. 1998, Hepatitis C, Lancet, 351(9099), pp. 351-355.

Diebold, S. S., Kaisho, T., Hemmi, H., Akira, S., Reis e Sousa 2004, Innate antiviral responses by means of TLR7-mediated recognition of single-stranded RNA, Science, 303(5663), pp. 1529-1531.

Dolganiuc, A., Norkina, O., Kodys, K., Catalano, D., Bakis, G., Marshall, C., Mandrekar, P., Szabo, G. 2007, Viral and host factors induce macrophage activation and loss of toll-like receptor tolerance in chronic HCV infection, Gastroenterology, 133(5), pp. 1627-1636.

Dolganiuc, A., Oak, S., Kodys, K., Golenbock, D. T., Finberg, R. W., Kurt-Jones, E., Szabo, G. 2004, Hepatitis C core and nonstructural 3 proteins trigger toll-like receptor 2-mediated pathways and inflammatory activation, Gastroenterology, 127(5), pp. 1513-1524.

Duesberg, U., von dem, B. A., Kirschning, C., Miyake, K., Sauerbruch, T., Spengler, U. 2002, Cell activation by synthetic lipopeptides of the hepatitis C virus (HCV)--core protein is mediated by toll like receptors (TLRs) 2 and 4, Immunol.Lett., 84(2), pp. 89-95.

Epstein, J., Eichbaum, Q., Sheriff, S., Ezekowitz, R. A. 1996, The collectins in innate immunity, Curr.Opin.Immunol., 8(1), pp. 29-35.

Eyre, N. S., Phillips, R. J., Bowden, S., Yip, E., Dewar, B., Locarnini, S. A., Beard, M. R. 2009, Hepatitis B virus and hepatitis C virus interaction in Huh-7 cells, J.Hepatol., 51(3), pp. 446-457.

Fearon, D. T., Locksley, R. M. 1996, The instructive role of innate immunity in the acquired immune response, Science, 272(5258), pp. 50-53.

Feldmann, G., Nischalke, H. D., Nattermann, J., Banas, B., Berg, T., Teschendorf, C., Schmiegel, W., Duhrsen, U., Halangk, J., Iwan, A., Sauerbruch, T., Caselmann, W. H., Spengler, U. 2006, Induction of interleukin-6 by hepatitis C virus core protein in hepatitis C-associated mixed cryoglobulinemia and B-cell non-Hodgkin's lymphoma, Clin.Cancer Res., 12(15), pp. 4491-4498.

Foy, E., Li, K., Sumpter, R., Jr., Loo, Y. M., Johnson, C. L., Wang, C., Fish, P. M., Yoneyama, M., Fujita, T., Lemon, S. M., Gale, M., Jr. 2005, Control of antiviral defenses through hepatitis C virus disruption of retinoic acid-inducible gene-I signaling, Proc.Natl.Acad.Sci.U.S.A, 102(8), pp. 2986-2991.

Foy, E., Li, K., Wang, C., Sumpter, R., Jr., Ikeda, M., Lemon, S. M., Gale, M., Jr. 2003, Regulation of interferon regulatory factor-3 by the hepatitis C virus serine protease, Science, 300(5622), pp. 1145-1148.

Frese, M., Pietschmann, T., Moradpour, D., Haller, O., Bartenschlager, R. 2001, Interferon-alpha inhibits hepatitis C virus subgenomic RNA replication by an MxA-independent pathway, J.Gen.Virol., 82(Pt 4), pp. 723-733.

Frese, M., Schwarzle, V., Barth, K., Krieger, N., Lohmann, V., Mihm, S., Haller, O., Bartenschlager, R. 2002, Interferon-gamma inhibits replication of subgenomic and genomic hepatitis C virus RNAs, Hepatology, 35(3), pp. 694-703.

Gale, M., Jr., Blakely, C. M., Kwieciszewski, B., Tan, S. L., Dossett, M., Tang, N. M., Korth, M. J., Polyak, S. J., Gretch, D. R., Katze, M. G. 1998, Control of PKR protein kinase by hepatitis C virus nonstructural 5A protein: molecular mechanisms of kinase regulation, Mol.Cell Biol., 18(9), pp. 5208-5218.

Gale, M., Jr., Kwieciszewski, B., Dossett, M., Nakao, H., Katze, M. G. 1999, Antiapoptotic and oncogenic potentials of hepatitis C virus are linked to interferon resistance by viral repression of the PKR protein kinase, J.Virol., 73(8), pp. 6506-6516.

Guidotti, L. G., Guilhot, S., Chisari, F. V. 1994, Interleukin-2 and alpha/beta interferon down-regulate hepatitis B virus gene expression in vivo by tumor necrosis factor-dependent and -independent pathways, J.Virol., 68(3), pp. 1265-1270.

Guidotti, L. G., Ishikawa, T., Hobbs, M. V., Matzke, B., Schreiber, R., Chisari, F. V. 1996, Intracellular inactivation of the hepatitis B virus by cytotoxic T lymphocytes, Immunity., 4(1), pp. 25-36.

Guo, H., Jiang, D., Ma, D., Chang, J., Dougherty, A. M., Cuconati, A., Block, T. M., Guo, J. T. 2009, Activation of pattern recognition receptor-mediated innate immunity inhibits the replication of hepatitis B virus in human hepatocyte-derived cells, J.Virol., 83(2), pp. 847-858.

Hadziyannis, S. J. 1997, Review: hepatitis delta, J.Gastroenterol.Hepatol., 12(4), pp. 289-298.

Hartwig, D., Schoeneich, L., Greeve, J., Schutte, C., Dorn, I., Kirchner, H., Hennig, H. 2004, Interferon-alpha stimulation of liver cells enhances hepatitis delta virus RNA editing in early infection, J.Hepatol., 41(4), pp. 667-672.

Hayashi, P. H., Zeldis, J. B. 1993, Molecular biology of viral hepatitis and hepatocellular carcinoma, Compr.Ther., 19(5), pp. 188-196.

Heim, M. H., Moradpour, D., Blum, H. E. 1999, Expression of hepatitis C virus proteins inhibits signal transduction through the Jak-STAT pathway, J.Virol., 73(10), pp. 8469-8475.

Helbig, K. J., Lau, D. T., Semendric, L., Harley, H. A., Beard, M. R. 2005, Analysis of ISG expression in chronic hepatitis C identifies viperin as a potential antiviral effector, Hepatology, 42(3), pp. 702-710.

Honda, K., Taniguchi, T. 2006, IRFs: master regulators of signalling by Toll-like receptors and cytosolic pattern-recognition receptors, Nat.Rev.Immunol., 6(9), pp. 644-658.

Hoesel, M., Quasdorff, M., Wiegmann, K., Webb, D., Zedler, U., Broxtermann, M., Tedjokusumo, R., Esser, K., Arzberger, S., Kirschning, C. J., Langenkamp, A., Falk, C., Buning, H., Rose-John, S., Protzer, U. 2009b, Not interferon, but interleukin-6 controls early gene expression in hepatitis B virus infection, Hepatology, 50(6), pp. 1773-1782.

Hui, D. J., Bhasker, C. R., Merrick, W. C., Sen, G. C. 2003, Viral stress-inducible protein p56 inhibits translation by blocking the interaction of eIF3 with the ternary complex eIF2.GTP.Met-tRNAi, J.Biol.Chem., 278(41), pp. 39477-39482.

Isogawa, M., Robek, M. D., Furuichi, Y., Chisari, F. V. 2005, Toll-like receptor signaling inhibits hepatitis B virus replication in vivo, J.Virol., 79(11), pp. 7269-7272.

Jacobson, I. M., McHutchison, J. G., Dusheiko, G., Di Bisceglie, A. M., Reddy, K. R., Bzowej, N. H., Marcellin, P., Muir, A. J., Ferenci, P., Flisiak, R., George, J., Rizzetto, M., Shouval, D., Sola, R., Terg, R. A., Yoshida, E. M., Adda, N., Bengtsson, L., Sankoh, A. J., Kieffer, T. L., George, S., Kauffman, R. S., Zeuzem, S. 2011, Telaprevir for previously untreated chronic hepatitis C virus infection, N.Engl.J.Med., 364(25), pp. 2405-2416.

Jurk, M., Heil, F., Vollmer, J., Schetter, C., Krieg, A. M., Wagner, H., Lipford, G., Bauer, S. 2002, Human TLR7 or TLR8 independently confer responsiveness to the antiviral compound R-848, Nat.Immunol., 3(6), p. 499.

Kimura, K., Kakimi, K., Wieland, S., Guidotti, L. G., Chisari, F. V. 2002, Activated intrahepatic antigen-presenting cells inhibit hepatitis B virus replication in the liver of transgenic mice, J.Immunol., 169(9), pp. 5188-5195.

Knolle, P. A., Gerken, G. 2000, Local control of the immune response in the liver, Immunol.Rev., 174, pp. 21-34.

Lee, J., Wu, C. C., Lee, K. J., Chuang, T. H., Katakura, K., Liu, Y. T., Chan, M., Tawatao, R., Chung, M., Shen, C., Cottam, H. B., Lai, M. M., Raz, E., Carson, D. A. 2006, Activation of anti-hepatitis C virus responses via Toll-like receptor 7, Proc.Natl.Acad.Sci.U.S.A, 103(6), pp. 1828-1833.

Li, K., Foy, E., Ferreon, J. C., Nakamura, M., Ferreon, A. C., Ikeda, M., Ray, S. C., Gale, M., Jr., Lemon, S. M. 2005, Immune evasion by hepatitis C virus NS3/4A protease-mediated cleavage of the Toll-like receptor 3 adaptor protein TRIF, Proc.Natl.Acad.Sci.U.S.A, 102(8), pp. 2992-2997.

Liaw, Y. F., Tsai, S. L., Chang, J. J., Sheen, I. S., Chien, R. N., Lin, D. Y., Chu, C. M. 1994, Displacement of hepatitis B virus by hepatitis C virus as the cause of continuing chronic hepatitis, Gastroenterology, 106(4), pp. 1048-1053.

Lin, W., Choe, W. H., Hiasa, Y., Kamegaya, Y., Blackard, J. T., Schmidt, E. V., Chung, R. T. 2005, Hepatitis C virus expression suppresses interferon signaling by degrading STAT1, Gastroenterology, 128(4), pp. 1034-1041.

Lin, W., Kim, S. S., Yeung, E., Kamegaya, Y., Blackard, J. T., Kim, K. A., Holtzman, M. J., Chung, R. T. 2006, Hepatitis C virus core protein blocks interferon signaling by interaction with the STAT1 SH2 domain, J.Virol., 80(18), pp. 9226-9235.

Lindenbach, B. D., Evans, M. J., Syder, A. J., Wolk, B., Tellinghuisen, T. L., Liu, C. C., Maruyama, T., Hynes, R. O., Burton, D. R., McKeating, J. A., Rice, C. M. 2005, Complete replication of hepatitis C virus in cell culture, Science, 309(5734), pp. 623-626.

Malakhov, M. P., Malakhova, O. A., Kim, K. I., Ritchie, K. J., Zhang, D. E. 2002, UBP43 (USP18) specifically removes ISG15 from conjugated proteins, J.Biol.Chem., 277(12), pp. 9976-9981.

Manns, M. P., McHutchison, J. G., Gordon, S. C., Rustgi, V. K., Shiffman, M., Reindollar, R., Goodman, Z. D., Koury, K., Ling, M., Albrecht, J. K. 2001, Peginterferon alfa-2b plus ribavirin compared with interferon alfa-2b plus ribavirin for initial treatment of chronic hepatitis C: a randomised trial, Lancet, 358(9286), pp. 958-965.

McClary, H., Koch, R., Chisari, F. V., Guidotti, L. G. 2000, Relative sensitivity of hepatitis B virus and other hepatotropic viruses to the antiviral effects of cytokines, J.Virol., 74(5), pp. 2255-2264.

McCormick, C. J., Challinor, L., Macdonald, A., Rowlands, D. J., Harris, M. 2004, Introduction of replication-competent hepatitis C virus transcripts using a tetracycline-regulable baculovirus delivery system, J.Gen.Virol., 85(Pt 2), pp. 429-439.

McNair, A. N., Cheng, D., Monjardino, J., Thomas, H. C., Kerr, I. M. 1994, Hepatitis delta virus replication in vitro is not affected by interferon-alpha or -gamma despite intact cellular responses to interferon and dsRNA, J.Gen.Virol., 75 (Pt 6), pp. 1371-1378.

Medzhitov, R. 2001, Toll-like receptors and innate immunity, Nat.Rev.Immunol., 1(2), pp. 135-145.

Medzhitov, R., Janeway, C., Jr. 2000, Innate immune recognition: mechanisms and pathways, Immunol.Rev., 173, pp. 89-97.

Mota, S., Mendes, M., Freitas, N., Penque, D., Coelho, A. V., Cunha, C. 2009, Proteome analysis of a human liver carcinoma cell line stably expressing hepatitis delta virus ribonucleoproteins, J.Proteomics., 72(4), pp. 616-627.

Mota, S., Mendes, M., Penque, D., Coelho, A. V., Cunha, C. 2008, Changes in the proteome of Huh7 cells induced by transient expression of hepatitis D virus RNA and antigens, J.Proteomics., 71(1), pp. 71-79.

Nakano, T., Shapiro, C. N., Hadler, S. C., Casey, J. L., Mizokami, M., Orito, E., Robertson, B. H. 2001, Characterization of hepatitis D virus genotype III among Yucpa Indians in Venezuela, J.Gen.Virol., 82(Pt 9), pp. 2183-2189.

Park, C. Y., Oh, S. H., Kang, S. M., Lim, Y. S., Hwang, S. B. 2009, Hepatitis delta virus large antigen sensitizes to TNF-alpha-induced NF-kappaB signaling, Mol.Cells, 28(1), pp. 49-55.

Pasquetto, V., Wieland, S. F., Uprichard, S. L., Tripodi, M., Chisari, F. V. 2002, Cytokine-sensitive replication of hepatitis B virus in immortalized mouse hepatocyte cultures, J.Virol., 76(11), pp. 5646-5653.

Pasquinelli, C., Shoenberger, J. M., Chung, J., Chang, K. M., Guidotti, L. G., Selby, M., Berger, K., Lesniewski, R., Houghton, M., Chisari, F. V. 1997, Hepatitis C virus core and E2 protein expression in transgenic mice, Hepatology, 25(3), pp. 719-727.

Perrault, M., Pecheur, E. I. 2009, The hepatitis C virus and its hepatic environment: a toxic but finely tuned partnership, Biochem.J., 423(3), pp. 303-314.

Pflugheber, J., Fredericksen, B., Sumpter, R., Jr., Wang, C., Ware, F., Sodora, D. L., Gale, M., Jr. 2002, Regulation of PKR and IRF-1 during hepatitis C virus RNA replication, Proc.Natl.Acad.Sci.U.S.A, 99(7), pp. 4650-4655.

Poordad, F., McCone, J., Jr., Bacon, B. R., Bruno, S., Manns, M. P., Sulkowski, M. S., Jacobson, I. M., Reddy, K. R., Goodman, Z. D., Boparai, N., DiNubile, M. J., Sniukiene, V., Brass, C. A., Albrecht, J. K., Bronowicki, J. P. 2011, Boceprevir for untreated chronic HCV genotype 1 infection, N.Engl.J.Med., 364(13), pp. 1195-1206.

Preiss, S., Thompson, A., Chen, X., Rodgers, S., Markovska, V., Desmond, P., Visvanathan, K., Li, K., Locarnini, S., Revill, P. 2008, Characterization of the innate immune signalling pathways in hepatocyte cell lines, J.Viral Hepat., 15(12), pp. 888-900.

Pugnale, P., Pazienza, V., Guilloux, K., Negro, F. 2009, Hepatitis delta virus inhibits alpha interferon signaling, Hepatology, 49(2), pp. 398-406.

Racanelli, V., Rehermann, B. 2006, The liver as an immunological organ, Hepatology, 43(2 Suppl 1), p. S54-S62.

Ritchie, K. J., Zhang, D. E. 2004, ISG15: the immunological kin of ubiquitin, Semin.Cell Dev.Biol., 15(2), pp. 237-246.

Rizzetto, M., Canese, M. G., Arico, S., Crivelli, O., Trepo, C., Bonino, F., Verme, G. 1977, Immunofluorescence detection of new antigen-antibody system (delta/anti-delta) associated to hepatitis B virus in liver and in serum of HBsAg carriers, Gut, 18(12), pp. 997-1003.

Rizzetto, M., Hoyer, B., Canese, M. G., Shih, J. W., Purcell, R. H., Gerin, J. L. 1980, delta Agent: association of delta antigen with hepatitis B surface antigen and RNA in serum of delta-infected chimpanzees, Proc.Natl.Acad.Sci.U.S.A, 77(10), pp. 6124-6128.

Saito, T., Hirai, R., Loo, Y. M., Owen, D., Johnson, C. L., Sinha, S. C., Akira, S., Fujita, T., Gale, M., Jr. 2007, Regulation of innate antiviral defenses through a shared repressor domain in RIG-I and LGP2, Proc.Natl.Acad.Sci.U.S.A, 104(2), pp. 582-587.

Sato, K., Ishikawa, T., Okumura, A., Yamauchi, T., Sato, S., Ayada, M., Matsumoto, E., Hotta, N., Oohashi, T., Fukuzawa, Y., Kakumu, S. 2007, Expression of Toll-like receptors in chronic hepatitis C virus infection, J.Gastroenterol.Hepatol., 22(10), pp. 1627-1632.

Schott, E., Witt, H., Neumann, K., Taube, S., Oh, D. Y., Schreier, E., Vierich, S., Puhl, G., Bergk, A., Halangk, J., Weich, V., Wiedenmann, B., Berg, T. 2007, A Toll-like receptor 7 single nucleotide polymorphism protects from advanced inflammation and fibrosis in male patients with chronic HCV-infection, J.Hepatol., 47(2), pp. 203-211.

Schuttler, C. G., Fiedler, N., Schmidt, K., Repp, R., Gerlich, W. H., Schaefer, S. 2002, Suppression of hepatitis B virus enhancer 1 and 2 by hepatitis C virus core protein, J.Hepatol., 37(6), pp. 855-862.

Sikora, D., Greco-Stewart, V. S., Miron, P., Pelchat, M. 2009, The hepatitis delta virus RNA genome interacts with eEF1A1, p54(nrb), hnRNP-L, GAPDH and ASF/SF2, Virology, 390(1), pp. 71-78.

Silverman, R. H. 1994, Fascination with 2-5A-dependent RNase: a unique enzyme that functions in interferon action, J.Interferon Res., 14(3), pp. 101-104.

Su, A. I., Pezacki, J. P., Wodicka, L., Brideau, A. D., Supekova, L., Thimme, R., Wieland, S., Bukh, J., Purcell, R. H., Schultz, P. G., Chisari, F. V. 2002, Genomic analysis of the host response to hepatitis C virus infection, Proc.Natl.Acad.Sci.U.S.A, 99(24), pp. 15669-15674.

Sumpter, R., Jr., Loo, Y. M., Foy, E., Li, K., Yoneyama, M., Fujita, T., Lemon, S. M., Gale, M., Jr. 2005, Regulating intracellular antiviral defense and permissiveness to hepatitis C virus RNA replication through a cellular RNA helicase, RIG-I, J.Virol., 79(5), pp. 2689-2699.

Sun, Z., Wada, T., Maemura, K., Uchikura, K., Hoshino, S., Diehl, A. M., Klein, A. S. 2003, Hepatic allograft-derived Kupffer cells regulate T cell response in rats, Liver Transpl., 9(5), pp. 489-497.

Suzuki, F., Arase, Y., Suzuki, Y., Tsubota, A., Akuta, N., Hosaka, T., Someya, T., Kobayashi, M., Saitoh, S., Ikeda, K., Kobayashi, M., Matsuda, M., Takagi, K., Satoh, J., Kumada, H. 2004, Single nucleotide polymorphism of the MxA gene promoter influences the response to interferon monotherapy in patients with hepatitis C viral infection, J.Viral Hepat., 11(3), pp. 271-276.

Takeda, K., Akira, S. 2005, Toll-like receptors in innate immunity, Int.Immunol., 17(1), pp. 1-14.

Taylor, D. R., Puig, M., Darnell, M. E., Mihalik, K., Feinstone, S. M. 2005, New antiviral pathway that mediates hepatitis C virus replicon interferon sensitivity through ADAR1, J.Virol., 79(10), pp. 6291-6298.

Taylor, D. R., Shi, S. T., Romano, P. R., Barber, G. N., Lai, M. M. 1999, Inhibition of the interferon-inducible protein kinase PKR by HCV E2 protein, Science, 285(5424), pp. 107-110.

Terenzi, F., Pal, S., Sen, G. C. 2005, Induction and mode of action of the viral stress-inducible murine proteins, P56 and P54, Virology, 340(1), pp. 116-124.

Thompson, A. J., Colledge, D., Rodgers, S., Wilson, R., Revill, P., Desmond, P., Mansell, A., Visvanathan, K., Locarnini, S. 2009, Stimulation of the interleukin-1 receptor and Toll-like receptor 2 inhibits hepatitis B virus replication in hepatoma cell lines in vitro, Antivir.Ther., 14(6), pp. 797-808.

Vilasco, M., Larrea, E., Vitour, D., Dabo, S., Breiman, A., Regnault, B., Riezu, J. I., Eid, P., Prieto, J., Meurs, E. F. 2006, The protein kinase IKKepsilon can inhibit HCV expression independently of IFN and its own expression is downregulated in HCV-infected livers, Hepatology, 44(6), pp. 1635-1647.

Visvanathan, K., Skinner, N. A., Thompson, A. J., Riordan, S. M., Sozzi, V., Edwards, R., Rodgers, S., Kurtovic, J., Chang, J., Lewin, S., Desmond, P., Locarnini, S. 2007, Regulation of Toll-like receptor-2 expression in chronic hepatitis B by the precore protein, Hepatology, 45(1), pp. 102-110.

Wakita, T., Pietschmann, T., Kato, T., Date, T., Miyamoto, M., Zhao, Z., Murthy, K., Habermann, A., Krausslich, H. G., Mizokami, M., Bartenschlager, R., Liang, T. J. 2005, Production of infectious hepatitis C virus in tissue culture from a cloned viral genome, Nat.Med., 11(7), pp. 791-796.

Wang, B., Trippler, M., Pei, R., Lu, M., Broering, R., Gerken, G., Schlaak, J. F. 2009a, Toll-like receptor activated human and murine hepatic stellate cells are potent regulators of hepatitis C virus replication, J.Hepatol., 51(6), pp. 1037-1045.

Wang, C., Pflugheber, J., Sumpter, R., Jr., Sodora, D. L., Hui, D., Sen, G. C., Gale, M., Jr. 2003, Alpha interferon induces distinct translational control programs to suppress hepatitis C virus RNA replication, J.Virol., 77(7), pp. 3898-3912.

Wang, N., Liang, Y., Devaraj, S., Wang, J., Lemon, S. M., Li, K. 2009b, Toll-like receptor 3 mediates establishment of an antiviral state against hepatitis C virus in hepatoma cells, J.Virol., 83(19), pp. 9824-9834.

Wedemeyer, H., Manns, M. P. 2010, Epidemiology, pathogenesis and management of hepatitis D: update and challenges ahead, Nat.Rev.Gastroenterol.Hepatol., 7(1), pp. 31-40.

Wieland, S. F., Eustaquio, A., Whitten-Bauer, C., Boyd, B., Chisari, F. V. 2005, Interferon prevents formation of replication-competent hepatitis B virus RNA-containing nucleocapsids, Proc.Natl.Acad.Sci.U.S.A, 102(28), pp. 9913-9917.

Wieland, S. F., Spangenberg, H. C., Thimme, R., Purcell, R. H., Chisari, F. V. 2004a, Expansion and contraction of the hepatitis B virus transcriptional template in infected chimpanzees, Proc.Natl.Acad.Sci.U.S.A, 101(7), pp. 2129-2134.

Williams, V., Brichler, S., Radjef, N., Lebon, P., Goffard, A., Hober, D., Fagard, R., Kremsdorf, D., Deny, P., Gordien, E. 2009, Hepatitis delta virus proteins repress hepatitis B virus enhancers and activate the alpha/beta interferon-inducible MxA gene, J.Gen.Virol., 90(Pt 11), pp. 2759-2767.

Wu, J., Lu, M., Meng, Z., Trippler, M., Broering, R., Szczeponek, A., Krux, F., Dittmer, U., Roggendorf, M., Gerken, G., Schlaak, J. F. 2007a, Toll-like receptor-mediated control of HBV replication by nonparenchymal liver cells in mice, Hepatology, 46(6), pp. 1769-1778.

Wu, J., Meng, Z., Jiang, M., Pei, R., Trippler, M., Broering, R., Bucchi, A., Sowa, J. P., Dittmer, U., Yang, D., Roggendorf, M., Gerken, G., Lu, M., Schlaak, J. F. 2008, Hepatitis B virus suppresses toll-like receptor-mediated innate immune responses in murine parenchymal and nonparenchymal liver cells, Hepatology.

Wu, J., Meng, Z., Jiang, M., Zhang, E., Trippler, M., Broering, R., Bucchi, A., Krux, F., Dittmer, U., Yang, D., Roggendorf, M., Gerken, G., Lu, M., Schlaak, J. F. 2009, Toll-like receptor-induced innate immune responses in non-parenchymal liver cells are cell type-specific, Immunology.

Wu, M., Xu, Y., Lin, S., Zhang, X., Xiang, L., Yuan, Z. 2007b, Hepatitis B virus polymerase inhibits the interferon-inducible MyD88 promoter by blocking nuclear translocation of Stat1, J.Gen.Virol., 88(Pt 12), pp. 3260-3269.

Xia, C., Lu, M., Zhang, Z., Meng, Z., Zhang, Z., Shi, C. 2008, TLRs antiviral effect on hepatitis B virus in HepG2 cells, J.Appl.Microbiol., 105(5), pp. 1720-1727.

Xu, Y., Kock, J., Lu, Y., Yang, D., Lu, M., Zhao, X. 2011, Suppression of hepatitis B virus replication in Tupaia hepatocytes by tumor necrosis factor alpha of Tupaia belangeri, Comp Immunol.Microbiol.Infect.Dis..

Yoneyama, M., Kikuchi, M., Natsukawa, T., Shinobu, N., Imaizumi, T., Miyagishi, M., Taira, K., Akira, S., Fujita, T. 2004, The RNA helicase RIG-I has an essential function in double-stranded RNA-induced innate antiviral responses, Nat.Immunol., 5(7), pp. 730-737.

Zarski, J. P., Bohn, B., Bastie, A., Pawlotsky, J. M., Baud, M., Bost-Bezeaux, F., Tran van, N. J., Seigneurin, J. M., Buffet, C., Dhumeaux, D. 1998, Characteristics of patients with dual infection by hepatitis B and C viruses, J.Hepatol., 28(1), pp. 27-33.

Zeuzem, S., Andreone, P., Pol, S., Lawitz, E., Diago, M., Roberts, S., Focaccia, R., Younossi, Z., Foster, G. R., Horban, A., Ferenci, P., Nevens, F., Mullhaupt, B., Pockros, P., Terg, R., Shouval, D., van, H. B., Weiland, O., Van, H. R., De, M. S., Luo, D., Boogaerts, G., Polo, R., Picchio, G., Beumont, M. 2011, Telaprevir for retreatment of HCV infection, N.Engl.J.Med., 364(25), pp. 2417-2428.

Zhang, X., Meng, Z., Qiu, S., Xu, Y., Yang, D., Schlaak, J. F., Roggendorf, M., Lu, M. 2009, Lipopolysaccharide-induced innate immune responses in primary hepatocytes downregulates woodchuck hepatitis virus replication via interferon-independent pathways, Cell Microbiol., 11(11), pp. 1624-1637.

Zhong, J., Gastaminza, P., Cheng, G., Kapadia, S., Kato, T., Burton, D. R., Wieland, S. F., Uprichard, S. L., Wakita, T., Chisari, F. V. 2005, Robust hepatitis C virus infection in vitro, Proc.Natl.Acad.Sci.U.S.A, 102(26), pp. 9294-9299.

Zhou, A., Paranjape, J., Brown, T. L., Nie, H., Naik, S., Dong, B., Chang, A., Trapp, B., Fairchild, R., Colmenares, C., Silverman, R. H. 1997, Interferon action and apoptosis are defective in mice devoid of 2',5'-oligoadenylate-dependent RNase L, EMBO J., 16(21), pp. 6355-6363.

3

Immunopathogenesis and Immunotherapy for Viral Hepatitis

Yukihiro Shimizu
Gastoenterology Unit, Takaoka City Hospital, Toyama, Japan

1. Introduction

Neither hepatitis B virus (HBV) nor hepatitis C virus (HCV) is cytopathic, and hepatitis is caused by the host immune response against virus-related peptides expressed on hepatocytes in conjunction with human leukocyte antigens (HLA). In acute self-limiting hepatitis, a broad immune response occurs that is strong enough to eradicate the virus or suppress viral replication (Rehermann, 1996). However, there are many mechanisms that hamper the antiviral immune response leading to persistent infection. To develop an optimal strategy to stimulate antiviral immune response with therapeutic potential, extensive analyses of immune mechanisms for successful viral eradication and immunosuppressive mechanisms induced by viral infection during persistent infection are required. The first half of this chapter discusses these points, followed by a discussion of immunotherapeutic approaches in both animal models and humans in the second half.

2. Immunological response in viral infection

2.1 Acute viral hepatitis

Immunological analysis has been extensively performed in transgenic and chimpanzee models of acute HBV infection. In one model, transgenic mice, in which infectious HBV virions replicate in the liver with expression of all HBV-related antigens, were injected with HBsAg-specific cytotoxic T lymphocytes (CTLs) that had been induced in nontransgenic mice. The injected CTLs produced interferon (IFN)-γ and tumor necrosis factor (TNF)-α, which purged viral RNA and DNA without destroying infected hepatocytes (Guidotti et al., a 1996; Chisari, 1997; Guidotti et al., 2001). Importantly, this noncytolytic clearance of intracellular HBV is more efficient at controlling HBV replication than the killing of infected hepatocytes. In this sense, hepatitis is not only a harmful event but also represents an effective mechanism by which CTLs suppress HBV. It is important to note that in the HBV transgenic mouse model of acute hepatitis, administration of antibodies against the chemokines, IFN-γ-inducible protein (IP-10) and monokine induced by interferon-γ (Mig) reduced the recruitment of mostly Ag-nonspecific mononuclear cells into the liver that had been induced by cytokines and chemokines produced by injected CTLs, leading to a reduction in the severity of hepatitis without affecting the antiviral activity of the CTLs (Kakimi et al., 2001). These observations have important therapeutic implications, because suppression of Ag-nonspecific mononuclear cell recruitment may suppress hepatitis while retaining the antiviral function of the CTLs. Noncytolytic viral eradication can account for recovery from acute HBV infection in that most HBV is cleared from hepatocytes with only a fraction of the hepatocytes being destroyed. This was confirmed in a chimpanzee infection model; HBV DNA level was markedly decreased in the liver and blood of acutely infected chimpanzees before peak serum alanine aminotransferase (ALT) concentrations were reached (Guidotti et al., 1999), suggesting that this noncytopathic T cell effector mechanism results in early viral inhibition or eradication, whereas a cytopathic T cell effector mechanism would be required to eliminate the remaining virus by destroying infected hepatocytes.

In humans, the HBV-specific T cell response during incubation phase of acute hepatitis B has been analyzed extensively using HLA class I tetramer and cytokine staining (Webster et al., 2000). The data showed that maximal reduction in HBV DNA in the serum occurred before the peak of ALT elevation, again indicating that suppression of HBV replication occurs without hepatocyte injury. Moreover, infiltration of HBV-specific CD8$^+$ T cells into the liver has been observed several weeks before the peak of liver injury, suggesting that HBV-specific T cell infiltration occurs at an early stage of infection resulting in suppression of HBV replication. Thereafter, recruitment of mostly nonspecific cells induced by cytokines or chemokines produced by HBV-specific T cells contributes to significant liver damage.

The overall data from studies in mice, chimpanzees, and humans are essentially the same, and indicate that a sufficient T cell response to HBV at an early phase of infection is important for eradication of virus infection, and that an insufficient T cell response may lead to persistent viral infection.

The same is essentially true in acute HCV infection. Multispecific and vigorous CTL responses against HCV antigens are important for successful eradication of the virus. Moreover, a CD4$^+$ T cell response at an early stage of acute infection and persistence of the response are apparent in acute infection (Semmo et al., 2007). In contrast to acute HBV infection, the majority of patients with acute HCV infection progress to persistent infection, and the mechanisms underlying failure to eradicate the virus have been analyzed. The failure of CD4$^+$ T cell function is a key factor in HCV persistence and CD4$^+$ T cells from persistent infection do not produce Th1 cytokines, such as IFN-γ and IL-2, but produce IL-4 and IL-10, clearly distinct from those seen in patients with recovery (Tsai et al., 1997). Moreover, an early and strong Th1 response has been shown to play an important role in disease resolution. One possible mechanism explaining why the Th2 type CD4$^+$ T cell response is dominant in patients with persistent infection is a defective function of dendritic cells, possibly due to lack of IL-12 production (Fowler et al., 2003).

2.2 Antigen-specificity of T cell response in viral hepatitis

The antigen-specificity of the T cell response to HBV in acute hepatitis has been analyzed, and it is clear that acute viral hepatitis involves a vigorous CTL response to multiple epitopes in the viral nucleocapsid, envelope, and polymerase proteins, while these are not seen in patients with chronic hepatitis (Rehermann, 1996). Although multi-specificity of the CTL response is characteristic in acute hepatitis, there is known to be a hierarchy of epitope-specific CD8$^+$ T cell responses determined by cytokine production after peptide stimulation. In acute hepatitis B, CD8$^+$ T cell response to HBc18-27 (HLA-A2 restricted epitope) is dominant followed by the response to polymerase epitope (455 – 463), whereas envelope epitopes are always subdominant (Webster et al., 2001). The hierarchy is clearly distinct from that observed in chronic hepatitis, in which the $CD8^+$ T cell response to envelope epitope (183 - 191) is always dominant. Interestingly, chronic hepatitis patients with lower HBV DNA levels in the serum show greater responses to HBc18-27 than those with high HBV DNA. These findings imply that the T cell response to HBcAg is important for viral control, which is important for designing peptide vaccines for the treatment of chronic HBV infection.

In acute HCV infection, the CTL responses were directed against multiple viral epitopes, in particular within the structural (core) and nonstructural (NS) regions of the virus (NS3, NS4, and NS5), and the CTL frequencies were higher in patients with acute infection (Cucchiarini et al., 2000; Lechner et al., 2000) than in those who develop persistent infection. The hierarchy of HCV epitopes has not been analyzed extensively, but resolution of primary infection in the chimpanzee was shown to be associated with a dominant $CD4^+$ T cell response against epitopes including NS3 (GYKVLVLNPSV), suggesting the existence of an HCV epitope hierarchy (Shoukry et al., 2004).

2.3 Chronic hepatitis

In contrast to acute hepatitis, the T cell response to HBV is weak and is narrowly focused in chronically infected patients (Chisari et al., 1995), suggesting that it may be a cause of persistent infection.

HBV-specific helper and cytotoxic T lymphocytes (CTLs) are barely detectable in peripheral blood of patients with chronic hepatitis B (Ferrari et al., 1990), possibly due to exhaustion by high viral load or tolerance to HBV. Maini et al. (2000) reported that the number of HBV-specific T cells, detected using tetramers was the same in livers with low HBV DNA/ALT as in those with high HBV DNA/ALT. Hence, HBV-specific T cells recognize HBV antigens and carry out immune surveillance in the liver. Thus, they have an important role in controlling HBV replication in the liver without causing hepatic necroinflammation in low DNA/ALT anti-HBe^+ HBV carriers. It remains unknown why HBV-specific T cells fail to effectively control HBV replication in the liver with chronic hepatitis. However, recent advances in immunology have given some insight into the mechanism as described below.

In contrast to chronic HBV infection, CTL response against various HCV epitopes including core, envelope and NS regions can be detected in chronic HCV infection, especially in liver-infiltrating lymphocytes (Koziel et al, 1995). Although intrahepatic CTL response was shown associated with low viral load (Freeman et al, 2003), the CTL response is not enough to terminate HCV infection possibly due to the presence of immunosuppressive mechanisms similar to chronic HBV infection.

3. Immunosuppressive mechanisms responsible for persistent hepatitis virus infection

3.1 Regulatory T cells (Tregs)

Tregs expressing the forkhead family transcription factor, Foxp3, are specialized cells that exert negative control on a variety of physiological and pathological immune responses, resulting in maintenance of immunological self-tolerance (Miyara et al., 2011). They show diverse phenotypes, occurring in both $CD4^+$ and $CD8^+$ T cell subsets, and express CD25 (IL-2 receptor α chain) and/or cytotoxic T-lymphocyte antigen 4 (CTLA-4) in addition to Foxp3.

In HBV infection, HBeAg-positive patients with high HBV DNA levels in the serum showed elevated numbers of $CD4^+CD25^+$ Treg cells in the blood compared to patients with acute or chronic HCV infection (Xu et al., 2006). Significant accumulation of $CD4^+CD25^+FoxP3^+$ Treg cells in the liver was found in patients with chronic HBV infection. Moreover, patients with high viral load have a higher proportion of Tregs in the liver (Stoop et al., 2008), suggesting that intrahepatic Tregs suppress antiviral immune responses in the liver in chronic hepatitis B virus infection. In HCV infection, it has also been shown that a higher frequency of $CD4^+CD25^+$ regulatory T cells in the blood of chronically HCV-infected patients versus recovered or healthy individuals (Cabrera et al., 2004; Boettler et al., 2005) and the presence of $CD4^+FoxP3^+$ T cells in the liver of chronically HCV-infected patients (Sturm et al., 2010).

3.2 Programmed Death-1 (PD-1)

PD-1 is a surface receptor critical for the regulation of T cell function (Francisco et al., 2010; Fife et al., 2011). Binding to PD-1 by its ligands PD-L1 and PD-L2 results in the antigen-specific inhibition of T cell proliferation, cytokine production, and cytolytic function, leading to exhaustion of T cells. In the liver, PD-1 is expressed on lymphocytes; PD-L1 is expressed on lymphocytes, hepatocytes, and sinusoidal endothelial cells, and PD-L2 is expressed on Kupffer cells and DCs (Chen et al., 2010). HBeAg-positive patients with high HBV DNA levels in the serum showed increased PD-1 and CTLA-4 expression on HBV-specific $CD8^+$ T cells (Peng et al., 2011). Moreover, PD-1 expression on $CD4^+$ T cells is correlated positively with serum HBV DNA load in CHB patients (Nan et al., 2010). Intrahepatic HBV-specific $CD8^+$ T cells express higher levels of PD-1, and upregulation of intrahepatic PD-1/PD-L1 is associated with liver inflammation and ALT elevation (Fisicaro et al., 2010). Although the mechanism underlying the upregulation of PD-1 on $CD8^+$ T cells in the inflamed liver is unknown, signals from PD-1 inhibit HBV-specific T cells, resulting in insufficient antiviral responses leading to failure of viral control and persistent liver inflammation. Importantly, PD-1/PD-L1 blockade increased $CD8^+$ T cell proliferation and enhanced IFN-γ and IL-2 production by intrahepatic lymphocytes (Fisicaro et al., 2010). These findings suggest that inhibition of PD-1/PD-L1 may have therapeutic potential for the control of hepatitis B.

Similar to T cells in patients with chronic hepatitis B, circulating and intrahepatic HCV-specific $CD8^+$ T cells were found to express high levels of PD-1 (Golden-Mason et al., 2007), and PD-1 expression level in the liver is higher than that in peripheral blood. Increased expression of PD-1 is associated with $CD8^+$ T cell dysfunction, and functional restoration is achieved by blocking the signal from PD-1 (Penna et al., 2007). Recently, HCV core protein was shown to induce PD-1 and PD-L1 on T cells from healthy donors (Yao et al., 2007), indicating that immunosuppressive ability of HCV core protein is mediated by the upregulation of inhibitory molecules on T cells. Increased PD-1 expression on HCV-specific CTLs was reported to be significantly associated with poor response to antiviral therapy (Golden-Mason et al., 2008), and PD-L1 expression on DCs is increased during IFN-a treatment (Urbani et al., 2008), suggesting that PD-1/PD-L1 is associated with the efficacy of antiviral treatment. PD-1 is also expressed on Tregs in the liver, and the signal from PD-1 ligation provides an overall inhibitory signal to Tregs. PD-1 blockade enhanced IL-2-dependent proliferation of intrahepatic Tregs in response to HCV antigens and enhanced the inhibitory ability of Tregs ((Franceschini et al. 2009), suggesting that complex interactions determine the direction of antiviral immune response.

3.3 Interluekin-10 (IL-10)

Interleukin (IL)-10 is an important cytokine with anti-inflammatory properties, and is produced by activated monocytes/macrophages and T cell subsets, including Treg and Th1 cells (Sabat et al., 2010). Immunosuppression by IL-10 is associated with functional exhaustion of memory T cells in chronic lymphocytic choriomeningitis virus (LCMV) infection, and blockade of IL-10 receptors could terminate chronic LCMV infection (Ejrnaes et al., 2006). In chronic HBV infection, HBcAg stimulates the production of IL-10, which negatively regulates HBcAg-specific Th17 cell responses in CHB patients (Li et al., 2010).

In HCV infection, peripheral blood mononuclear cells produce IL-17, IFN-γ, IL-10, and TGF-β in response to NS4 protein of HCV, and neutralization of TGF-β or IL-10 significantly enhances NS4-specific IL-17 and IFN-γ production by T cells from HCV-infected patients (Rowan et al., 2008). Moreover, lipopolysaccharide and HCV core protein trigger IL-10 and TNF-α production from monocytes, but at much lower levels from monocytes in patients with self-limiting HCV infection (Martin-Blondel et al., 2008). These data indicate that HCV proteins induce IL-10 from monocytes in patients with chronic HCV infection, leading to suppression of antiviral immune response.

3.4 T-cell immunoglobulin and mucin domain-containing molecule-3 (Tim-3)

It has been reported that not all exhausted T cells show upregulation of PD-1 and downregulation of CD127 (IL-7 receptor), and blockade of the PD-1/PD-L1 signaling pathway does not always restore proliferation and cytokine production (Golden-Mason et al., 2009). Recently, another inhibitory molecule, Tim-3, has been reported. A high frequency of Tim3-expressing $CD4^+$ and $CD8^+$ T cells are found in chronic HBV infection, and the frequency of Tim-3^+ T cells was positively correlated with the severity of liver inflammation, and negatively correlated with plasma IFN-γ levels (Ju et al., 2009). Tim-3 was also highly expressed on $CD4^+$ and $CD8^+$ T cells in HCV infection, with the highest levels seen on HCV-specific CTLs. Tim-3 expression is associated with reduced Th1/Tc1 cytokine production, and blocking the Tim-3 – Tim-3 ligand interaction could enhance $CD4^+$ and $CD8^+$ T cell proliferation in response to HCV-specific antigens (Golden-Mason et al., 2009).

3.5 Dysfunction of DCs

DCs are specialized antigen-presenting cells that orchestrate immune responses. They stimulate innate and acquired immune responses, but also act as tolerogenic cells for immune responses in a variety of situations. In viral hepatitis, dysfunction of DCs from peripheral blood has been reported. In patients with chronic hepatitis B, maturation of DCs from peripheral blood of patients after incubation with cytokines is lower than that of normal subjects with lower expression of HLA-DR and costimulatory molecules in the former population (Wang et al., 2001), leading to low allostimulatory function of DCs from CHB patients. The mechanism of impairment of DC function in patients with chronic hepatitis B is unclear, but both HBV particles and purified HBsAg may have immunomodulatory capacity and may directly contribute to the dysfunction of myeloid DCs (Op den Brouw et al., 2009). Importantly, impaired function of monocyte-derived DCs from patients with CHB could be reversed by inhibiting viral replication with nucleoside analogs such as lamivudine (Beckebaum et al., 2003). Type 2 precursor plasmacytoid dendritic cells (pDCs), which are the most important cells in antiviral innate immunity, were also reported to have quantitative and qualitative impairment in patients with chronic HBV infection (Duan et al., 2004). Recently, HBV itself was shown to inhibit the functions of pDCs (Woltman et al., 2011). These data indicate that DCs in patients with chronic hepatitis B have impaired function leading to insufficient T cell response to HBV, which could be the mechanism responsible for persistent viral infection.

In chronic hepatitis C, DCs from patients also show impaired immunostimulatory function, which could be induced by HCV (Eksioglu et al., 2010) or NS4 protein (Takaki et al., 2010). Monocyte-derived DCs from HCV patients were shown to induce proliferation of $CD4^+CD25^+FoxP3^+$ regulatory T cells, which limit proliferation of HCV-specific T lymphocytes (Dolganiuc et al., 2008). DCs in HCV patients thus inhibit T cell responses via a variety of mechanisms.

4. Immunotherapy for viral hepatitis

Therapeutic strategies for terminating viral infection should be evaluated based on the mechanisms responsible for insufficient antiviral immunological mechanisms leading to persistent viral infection. Most immunotherapeutic approaches for viral hepatitis have been directed against hepatitis B. This is likely due to the availability of good animal models of persistent HBV infection, ready availability of HB vaccine and accumulation of basic immunological analyses. Previous animal studies and human trials are listed in Tables 1 and 2, respectively.

Peptide vaccination

Wang et al. 2010; A synthesized fusion peptide, consisting of HBcAg18-27 and HIV Tat49-57 adjuvanted with CpG ODN increased $CD3^+$, $CD4^+$ and $CD8^+$ cells and the production of IFN-γ and IL-2. Vaccination with the peptide reduced serum HBV DNA levels and decreased the expression levels of HBsAg and HBcAg in the livers of transgenic mice.

Protein vaccination

Akbar et al, 1997; HBV transgenic mice were treated with vaccine on the base of surface antigen in complete Freund's adjuvant once a month for 12 months. Most of the mice showed reduction of HBV DNA level and disappearance of HBeAg and HBsAg.

Menne et al, 2007; A combination of conventional vaccine on the base of the WHV large surface protein contained HBsAg with pre-S and clevudine significantly restored the T-cell response to Pre-S and S region in chronic WHV infection.

Miller at al, 2008; One hour post-infection with DHBV, DNA vaccine expressing DHBc and Pre-S/S and entecavir were given simultaneously and continued for 14 days. Ducks boosted with fowl poxvirus vectors expressing DHBc and Pre-S/S showed clearance of DHBV infection at a rate of 100%.

DNA immunization

Thermet et al, 2008; DNA vaccine encoding the DHBV large envelope and/or core protein was given 6 times with or without lamivudine in a DHBV model. Reduction of viremia and liver DHBV cccDNA was observed in 33% of ducks receiving DNA vaccine mono- or combination therapy. Seroconversion to anti-pre S was observed in 67% of ducks showing cccDNA clearance.

Encke et al, 2006; The combination of DNA vaccination encoding HCV core and mouse IL-2 breaks tolerance and activates previously tolerant T cells in an HCV transgenic mouse model.

DC immunization
Shimizu et al, 1998; Activated bone marrow-derived DCs were shown to break CTL tolerance to HBsAg in HBV transgenic mice.
Kimura et al, 2002; A single injection of an anti-CD40 agonistic monoclonal antibody into HBV transgenic mice induced noncytopathic inhibition of HBV replication, which was mediated by antiviral cytokines (IL-12 and TNF-α) produced by activated intrahepatic antigen-presenting cells.
Jiang et al, 2008; HBV transgenic mice were injected with HBV-specific peptide-pulsed DCs, and significant reductions in the serum HBsAg and HBV DNA concentrations were observed.
Díaz-Valdés et al, 2011; DCs, treated with peptide inhibitors of IL-10, induced strong anti-HCV T cell responses in HCV transgenic mice.
Cytokines and adjuvants
Cavanaugh et al, 1997; Recombinant IL-12 markedly inhibits HBV replication in the liver of HBV transgenic mice through its ability to induce IFN-γ.
Kakimi et al, 2000; A single injection of α-galactosylceramide that can activate Valpha14$^+$NK1.1$^+$T cells (NKT cells) abolished HBV replication in HBV transgenic mice.
Kimura et al, 2002; Injection of IL-18 into HBV transgenic mice inhibited HBV replication noncytopathically, which was mediated by activation of resident intrahepatic NK cells and NKT cells.
Gene therapy
Hong et al, 2011; Lentivectors expressing HBsAg and IgFc fusion Ag could effectively break immune tolerance and induced seroconversion to anti-HBs in HBsAg transgenic mice.

CpG ODN; CpG oligodeoxynucleotide, WHV; woodchuck hepatitis virus, DHBV; duck hepatitis B virus, cccDNA; covalently closed circular DNA, NKT; natural killer T

Table 1. Immunotherapeutic approaches for animal models of HBV and HCV infection.

Peptide vaccination
Heathcote et al, 1999; A vaccine with HBc18-27 peptide comprised of a T-helper cell epitope and two palmitic acid residues was administered to chronic hepatitis B (CHB) patients. Low levels of CTL activity were induced, but no significant changes in liver biochemistry or viral serology were observed.
Klade et al, 2008; A vaccine containing 7 relevant HCV T cell epitopes and the Th1 adjuvant poly-L-arginine, induced HCV-specific Th1/Tc1 responses in a subset of HCV patients not responding to or relapsing from standard therapy. However, only a minimal decrease in HCV viremia was induced by the vaccination.
Yutani et al, 2009; Vaccination with a peptide derived from HCV core protein induced both cellular and humoral responses in nearly all HCV patients with different HLA class I-A alleles, and reduced serum ALT and α-fetoprotein levels in 29% and 50% of patients, respectively.
Protein vaccination
Pol et al; 2001; Five intramuscular injections of 20μg of a preS2/S (GenHevac B) or S

(Recombivax) vaccine in CHB patients showed HBe/anti-HBe seroconversion in 13% and HBV DNA negativity in 16% of the treated patients.
Dahmen et al, 2002; Intradermal commercially available HBV vaccine and laimvudine in combination with IL-2 induced a significant antiviral response, leading to HBV DNA loss in the serum in two of five patients with chronic hepatitis B.
Klein et al, 2003; Oral administration of HBV envelope proteins (HBsAg+preS1+preS2) to CHB patients three times a week for 20 to 30 weeks induced histological improvement in 30% of the patients, HBeAg negativity in 26.3% and HBsAg-specific T cell proliferation in 78%.
Helvaci et al, 2003; Children with CHB were treated with IFN-α-2b monotherapy (9 months) or IFN-α-2b plus HBV pre-S2/S vaccine (0, 4, 24weeks). The patients who received the combination therapy showed a greater reduction in HBV DNA than those who received IFN-α-2b monotherapy.
Vandepapelière et al, 2007; In HBeAg-positive CHB patients, the combination with lamivudune and vaccine on the base of surface antigen with adjuvant did not improve the HBe seroconversion rate in comparison with lamivudine therapy alone.
Senturk et al, 2009; CHB patients who were treated with lamivudine and vaccine on the base of surface antigen showed sustained negativity of HBV DNA in 1/4 of the treated patients.
Al-Mahtab et al, 2010; CHB patients were treated with lamivudine and vaccine on the base of surface antigen (5 times) for 12 months. HBV DNA became undetectable in 64% of the patients, and was decreased in the remaining patients at the end of the combination therapy. No patients showed ALT elevation.

DNA immunization.

Mancini-Bourgine et al, 2004; DNA vaccine encoding HBV envelope protein induced an increase in HBV-specific IFN-γ-secreting T cells in patients with CHB, who had been nonresponders to conventional therapies, and HBV DNA levels were transiently decreased in 50% of vaccinated patients.
Mancini-Bourgine et al, 2006; DNA vaccine encoding PreS and S was administered to $HBeAg^{+}$ CHB patients with lamivudine breakthrough, and the patients developed IFN-γ-producing T cells specific for preS or S antigen. Two of 10 patients showed seroconversion to anti-HBe.
Alvarez-Lajonchere et al; 2009; A new vaccine, CIGB0230, consisting of a mixture of plasmid expressing HCV structural antigens and HCV recombinant core protein, Co.120 was intramuscularly administered 6 times within 20 weeks in patients with chronic HCV infection. The vaccination induced specific T cell proliferation and IFN-γ production in 73%. More than 40% of vaccinees showed improvement of liver histology, despite persistent detection of HCV RNA.

DC immunization

Chen et al, 2005; Peripheral blood-derived DCs, activated with GM-CSF and IL-4, were pulsed with HBsAg, and were administered subcutaneously twice in CHB patients. Both patients with normal and elevated ALT responded equally to DC vaccine and 53% of the patients showed induction of HBeAg negativity.

Luo et al, 2010; Activated DCs were generated from $CD14^+$ cells of PBL with GM-CSF and IL-4, and two peptides, HBcAg18-27 and PreS244-53, were loaded. Aliquots of $5x10^6$ to $3x10^7$ DCs were infused intravenously, and reinfusion was performed once or twice a month for 3 months. Undetectable HBV DNA was achieved in 46.3% and 3.13% of $HBeAg^-$ and $HBeAg^+$ patients, respectively. ALT normalization was observed in 69% of HBeAg- patients and in 30.5% of $HBeAg^+$ patients.

Gowans et al, 2010; Monocyte-derived DCs loaded with lipopeptides consisting of HCV-specific HLA-A2.1-restricted CTL epitopes, can induce HCV-specific $CD8^+$ T cell responses with IFN-γ production in PBL in HCV patients in whom conventional IFN-based therapy has failed. However, ALT levels were not elevated and viral load was not decreased.

Cytokines

Martin et al, 1993; Granulocyte macrophage-colony stimulating factor (GM-CSF) was safe and tolerable up to 1.0μg/kg body wt, and induced HBV DNA negativity in 4/8 patients with chronic HBV infection.

Wang et al, 2002; Combination therapy with GM-CSF (50μg) and vaccine on the base of surface antigen (10μg) (four intramuscular injections) significantly reduced serum HBV DNA in HBV carrier children.

Zeuzem et al, 2001; HBV DNA clearance was observed in 25% of CHB patients treated with a high dose of IL-12 (0.5μg/kg), and a reduction of >50% in HCV RNA level was observed in 53% of CHC patients treated with the same dose of IL-12.

Rigopoulou et al, 2005; The addition of IL-12 to lamivudine therapy stimulated T cell response to HBV with IFN-γ production. However, IL-12 was unable to suppress re-elevation of HBV DNA after cessation of lamivudine.

Szkaradkiewicz et al, 2005; Combination of IL-12 and IL-18 stimulated IFN-γ production by $CD4^+$ T cells isolated from peripheral blood of children with chronic hepatitis B in response to HBcAg, and the effect was greater than those observed with either cytokine alone.

Woltman et al, 2009; α-galactosylceramide was administered to patients with chronic HBV infection. It was poorly tolerated and showed no clear suppressive effect on serum HBV DNA or ALT levels.

Thymosin-α 1 (Talpha1)

Arase et al, 2003; The combination of Talpha1 and IFN-α for 24 weeks showed no statistically significant differences as compared with IFN-α monotherapy with respect to HBeAg seroconversion, changes in histology, normalization of ALT or loss of HBV DNA.

Iino et al, 2005; CHB patients were treated with Talpha1 for 24 weeks. At 12 months after cessation of therapy, 36.4% of patients treated with 1.6mg of Talpha1 achieved ALT normalization, 15% achieved HBV DNA clearance by transcription-mediated amplification, and 22.8% achieved clearance of HBeAg.

You et al, 2006; Efficacy of Talpha1 treatment was compared with IFN-α, and Talpha1 treatment was more effective in achieving ALT normalization and HBV DNA negativity at the end of the follow-up period than IFN-α.

Lee et al, 2008; The combination of Talpha1 and lamivudine did not show any additional antiviral effect compared with lamivudine monotherapy as determined by HBe seroconversion and the emergence of viral breakthrough. Zhang et al, 2009; A meta analysis demonstrated that combination therapy with lamivudine and Talpha1 yielded significantly higher rates of ALT normalization, virological response, and HBeAg seroconversion than lamivudine monotherapy. Poo et al, 2008; Patients with chronic HCV infection who had been nonresponders to prior IFN-α and ribavirin were treated with Talpha1, PEG-IFN α-2a, and ribavirin for 48 weeks. Twenty-four percent of the treated patients with genotype 1 achieved a sustained virological response.

GM-CSF; granulocyte macrophage-colony stimulating factor

Table 2. Immunotherapeutic trials for chronic HBV and HCV infection in humans

5. Immunotherapeutic approaches for viral hepatitis (Table 1 and 2)

Immunotherapeutic strategies for viral hepatitis include suppression of viral replication, induction of immune response to hepatitis virus, activation of nonspecific cells, and administration of cytokines with antiviral activity.

5.1 Suppression of viral replication

High viral load has been shown to suppress $CD4^+$ and $CD8^+$ T cells in addition to induction of Tregs, which could be reversed by antiviral therapy (Boni et al., 2001). Therefore, immunotherapy followed by restoration of virus-specific T cell response with antiviral therapy could be more efficient, especially in CHB.

5.2 Induction of immune response to hepatitis virus

5.2.1 Peptide immunization

A peptide vaccine containing highly immunogenic HBc18-27 has been developed and administered to CHB patients (Heathcote et al., 1999), but the results were disappointing because there was no induction of a significant antiviral T cell response. There have also been no reports of efficient peptide vaccination in HCV infection.

5.2.2 Protein immunization

In a model of HBV in transgenic mice, vaccine on the base of surface antigen in complete Freund's adjuvant once a month for 12 months induced reduction in HBV DNA, and the disappearance of HBeAg and HBsAg in most mice treated. Moreover, it is important to note that some mice developed anti-HBs in the sera (Akbar et al., 1997). However, several human trials with vaccine on the base of surface antigen showed limited efficacy if used as monotherapy.

Recently, HB vaccine containing not only S protein but also preS has been used with increased immunogenicity (Pol et al., 2001, Klein et al., 2003), or has been combined with lamivudine or IFN-α (Helvaci et al., 2003) leading to potential improvement of clinical efficacy. However, analysis on the T cell epitope hierarchy indicated that the most important epitope for viral control is HBc18-27, and not the HBsAg epitope in HLA-A2 patients

(Webster et al., 2001), suggesting the necessity of reconsidering antigen selection for vaccination that could lead to better viral control.

5.2.3 DNA immunization

Injection of plasmid DNA has been shown to strongly elicit both cellular and humoral immune responses, and is now known to be safe and well-tolerated both in mice and humans. In a model of duck hepatitis B virus infection, DNA vaccine encoding HBV large envelope and/or core protein was shown to induce reduction in not only viremia but also cccDNA in the liver in one third of ducks receiving DNA monotherapy or combination treatment along with lamivudine (Thermet et al., 2008). This finding is encouraging because clearance of cccDNA from the liver is the goal of treatment for HBV infection, but is difficult to achieve using IFN-α or nucleoside analogs. Clinical trials have also been performed in both HBV and HCV infection with some encouraging results (Table 2), which remain to be confirmed by future randomized large-scale trials.

5.2.4 DC immunization

DCs are specialized antigen-presenting cells that can induce strong immune responses in T and B cell. We have previously shown that activated bone marrow-derived DCs can break CTL tolerance to HBsAg in HBV transgenic mice (Shimizu et al., 1998). Thereafter, several immunotherapies with activated DCs have been applied in both animals and humans (Table 1 and 2). In a recent study performed in HBV transgenic mice, peptide-pulsed DCs were shown to significantly reduce the concentrations of serum HBsAg and HBV DNA (Jiang et al., 2003), indicating therapeutic potential in chronic HBV infection. Recently, DCs treated with peptide inhibitors of IL-10 were shown to induce strong anti-HCV T cell response in HCV transgenic mice (Díaz-Valdés et al., 2011), suggesting a strategy to augment the immunogenic function of DCs. Moreover, when intrahepatic antigen-presenting cells, including DCs, were activated by injection of an anti-CD40 agonistic antibody, HBV replication was inhibited by a noncytopathic mechanism possibly through production of antiviral cytokines such as TNF-α and IL-12 (Kimura et al., 2002a). Although no CTL response against HBV antigens was reported in this study, the in vivo activation of DCs could be an alternative way for inducing antiviral immune responses including possible activation of CTLs against HBV. In humans, injection of activated DCs loaded with HBV peptide or protein achieved a reduction in HBV DNA level in some patients (Chen et al., 2005, Luo et al., 2010). HBeAg negativity was achieved in more than half of the treated patients in one study (Chen et al., 2005). Although preparation of activated and mature DCs incurs financial costs and requires experienced researchers, immunotherapy with DCs is a promising method.

5.2.5 Natural Killer T (NKT) cells

A single injection of α-galactosylceramide abolished HBV replication by activating NKT cells in the liver in HBV transgenic mice (Kakimi et al., 2000). However, α-galactosylceramide was poorly tolerated in humans and showed no clear antiviral effect (Woltman et al., 2009), possibly due to smaller numbers of NKT cells in the human liver than in the mouse liver.

5.2.6 Cytokines and Thymosin-α1 (Talpha1)

Cytokines such as IL-12 (Cavanaugh et al., 1997) and IL-18 (Kimura et al., 2000b) were shown to inhibit HBV replication noncytopathically in HBV transgenic mice. In humans, GM-CSF (Martin et al., 1993, Wang et al., 2002) and IL-12 (Carreño et al., Zeuzem et al., 2001, Rigopoulou et al., 2005) have been used for treatment with some antiviral effects. They have been used as monotherapy or in combination with HB vaccine or lamivudine.

Talpha1, a synthetic 28-amino acid peptide, is able to enhance the Thl immune response and also exerts a direct antiviral mechanism of action. It has been used for the treatment of chronic HBV (Arase et al, 2003, Iino et al., 2005, You et al., 2006, Lee et al., 2008) and HCV (Poo et al., 2008) infection in humans, and showed antiviral effect with some efficacy. Although antiviral effect by the addition of Talpha1 to lamivudine or IFN-α therapy was controversial, a meta analysis demonstrated that the combination therapy with lamivudine and Talpha1 showed significantly higher rates of ALT normalization, virological response, and HBeAg seroconversion as compared with lamivudine monotherapy (Zhang et al., 2009). It is of note that HBeAg seroconversion rate was 45% in the combination group, which was significantly higher than that with lamivudine monotherapy (15%).

DCs
Akbar et al, 2010; DCs from peripheral blood and pulsed with HBsAg/HBcAg could induce HBsAg- and HBcAg-specific T cell proliferation in CHB patients.
PD-1
Nakamoto et al, 2009; CTLA-4 is preferentially expressed in PD-1$^+$ T cells from the liver with chronic HCV infection, and coexpression of CTLA-4 and PD-1 is associated with T cell dysfunction. Combined blockade of these molecules, but not blocking of either molecule, can reverse CD8$^+$ T cell exhaustion.
Ha et al, 2008; Blocking PD-1, CTLA-4 and IL-10 combined with therapeutic vaccination could synergistically enhance functional CD8$^+$ T cell response and improve viral control in chronically infected mice. Moreover, addition of stimulatory signals, such as IL-2, could further increase the efficacy of the therapy.
CD244
Raziorrouh et al, 2010; PD-1 and CD244 are highly coexpreesed on virus-specific CD8+ T cells in chronic HBV infection. Blocking signals through CD244 and its ligand CD48 could restore T cell dysfunction independent of the PD-1 pathway.
Tim-3
McMahan et al, 2010; Blockade of Tim-3 on human HCV-specific CTLs increased cytotoxicity against an HCVAg-expressing hepatocyte cell line that expresses HCV epitopes.
Golden-Mason et al, 2009; Tim-3 expression was increased on both CD4$^+$ and CD8$^+$ T cells in chronic hepatitis C infection, and PD-1/Tim-3 double positive T cells are accumulated in the liver with chronic hepatitis C. Blocking Tim-3/Tim-3 ligand induced T cell proliferation and IFN-γ production in response to HCV antigens.
Gene transfection
Zhang et al, 2010; Human T cells transduced with HCV TCR specific for HCV NS3 1071-1081 (HLA A2-restricted epitope) recognize the peptide and produced IFN-γ, IL-2 and TNF-α.

PD-1; programmed death-1, CTLA-4; cytotoxic T lymphocyte antigen-4, Tim-3; T-cell immunoglobulin and mucin domain-containing molecule-3

Table 3. Human basic research for improvement of immunotherapy for viral hepatitis.

Moreover, there have been several basic attempts to improve the efficacy of immunotherapy (Table 3). Among these reports, augmentation or restoration of T cell response by blocking the inhibitory signals have been extensively analyzed in vitro. It has been demonstrated that exhausted T cells express not only PD-1, but also CTLA-4 (Nakamoto et al., 2009), CD244 (Raziorrouch et al., 2010) or Tim-3 (Golden-Mason et al., 2009), and blocking of these molecules in combination could be better than blocking any single molecule to achieve full activation of the exhausted T cells.

6. Conclusion

There have been several attempts to apply immunotherapy for the control of chronic HBV and HCV infection, and some of the data are promising. Viral suppression, stimulation of antiviral immune response with cytokines, DNA or DC immunization and suppression of the immunoinhibitory signals must be combined to achieve desirable antiviral effects. Further studies are required to explore the best protocols and their most efficient combinations to become a promising and practical treatment.

7. References

Akbar, SM.; Kajino, K. Tanimoto, K. Kurose, K. Masumoto, T. Michitaka, K et al. (1997). *J. Hepatol,* Vol.26, No.1, (January 1997), pp. 131-137.

Akbar, SM.; Yoshida, O. Chen, S. Cesar, AJ. Abe, M. Matsuura, B et al. (2010). *Antivir Ther,* Vol.15, No.6, (2010), pp. 887-895.

Al-Mahtab M, Rahman S, Akbar SM, Khan SI, Uddin H, Karim F, et al. (2010). *Viral Immunol,* Vol.23, No.3, (June 2010), 335-338.

Alvarez-Lajonchere, L.; Shoukry, NH. Grá, B. Amador-Cañizares, Y. Helle, F. Bédard, N et al. (2009). *J Viral Hepat,* Vol.16, No.3, (October 2008), pp. 156-167.

Arase, Y.; Tsubota, A. Suzuki, Y. Suzuki, F. Kobayashi, M. Someya, T et al. (2003). *Intern Med,* Vol.42, No.10, (October 2003), pp. 941-946.

Barth, H.; Klein, R. Berg, PA. Wiedenmann, B. Hopf, U. & Berg, T. (2001). *Hepatogastroenterology,* Vol.48, No.38, (March-April 2001), pp. 553-555.

Beckebaum, S.; Cicinnati, VR. Zhang, X., Ferencik, S. Frilling, A. Grosse-Wilde, H. et al. (2003). *Immunology,* Vol.109, No.4, (August 2003), pp. 487-495.

Boettler, T.; Spangenberg, HC. Neumann-Haefelin, C. Panther, E. Urbani, S. Ferrari, C et al. (2005). *J Virol,* Vol.79, No.12, (Junuary 2005), pp. 7860-7867.

Boni, C.; Penna, A. Ogg, GS. Bertoletti, A. Pilli, M. Cavallo, C. et al. (2001). *Hepatology,* Vol.33, No.4, (April 2001), pp. 963-971.

Cabrera, R.; Tu, Z. Xu, Y. Firpi, RJ. Rosen, HR. Liu, C. et al. (2004). *Hepatology,* Vol.40, No.5, (November 2004), pp. 1062-1071.

Cavanaugh, VJ.; Guidotti, LG. & Chisari, FV. (1977). *J Virol,* Vol.71, No.4, (April 1997), pp. 3236-3243.

Chen, M.; Li, YG. Zhang, DZ. Wang, ZY. Zeng, WQ. Shi, XF. et al. (2005). *World J Gastroenterol,* Vol.11, No.12, (March 2005), pp. 1806-1808.

Chen, J; Wang, XM. Wu, XJ. Wang, Y. Zhao, H. Shen, B. et al. (2011). *Inflamm Res,* Vol.60, No.1, (July 2010), pp. 47-53.

Chisari, FV. & Ferrari, C. (1995). *Springer Semin Immunopathol,* (1995), Vol.17, No.2-3, pp. 261-281.

Chisari, FV. (1997). *J Clin Invest,* Vol.99, No.7, (April 1997), pp. 1472-1477.

Cucchiarini, M.; Kammer, AR. Grabscheid, B. Diepolder, HM. Gerlach, TJ. Grüner, N. et al. (2000). *Cell Immunol,* Vol.203, No.2, (August 2000), pp. 111-123.

Dahmen, A.; Herzog-Hauff, S. Böcher, WO. Galle, PR. & Löhr HF. (2002). *J Med Virol,* Vol.66, No.4, (Apr 2002), pp. 452-460.

Díaz-Valdés, N.; Manterola, L. Belsúe, V. Riezu-Boj, JI. Larrea, E. Echeverria, I. et al. (2011). *Hepatology,* Vol.53, No.1, (January 2011), pp.23-31.

Dolganiuc, A.; Paek, E. Kodys, K. Thomas, J. & Szabo, G. (2008). *Gastroenterology,* Vol.135, No.6. (December 2008), pp. 2119-2127.

Duan, XZ.; Wang, M. Li, HW. Zhuang, H. Xu, D. & Wang, FS. (2004). *J Clin Immunol,* Vol.24, No.6, (November 2004), pp. 637-646.

Ejrnaes M, Filippi CM, Martinic MM, Ling EM, Togher LM, Crotty S, et al. (2006). *J Exp Med,* Vol.203, No.11, (October 2006), pp. 2461-2472.

Eksioglu, EA.; Bess, JR. Zhu H. Xu Y. Dong, HJ. Elyar, J. et al. (2010). *J Viral Hepat,* Vol.17, No.11, (November 2010), pp. 757-769.

Encke, J.; Geissler, M. Stremmel, W. & Wands, JR. (2006). *Hum Vaccin,* Vol.2, No.2, (March 2006), pp. 78-83.

Ferrari, C.; Penna, A. Bertoletti, A. Valli, A. Antoni, AD. Giuberti, T. et al. (1990). *J Immunol,* Vol.45, No.10, (November 1990), pp. 3442-3449.

Fife, BT. & Pauken, KE. (2011). *Ann N Y Acad Sci,* Vol.1217, (January 2011), pp. 45-59.

Fisicaro, P; Valdatta, C. Massari, M. Loggi, E. Biasini, E. Sacchelli, L. et al. (2010). *Gastroenterology.* Vol.138, No.2, (September 2009), pp. 682-693, 693.e1-4.

Fowler, NL.; Torresi, J. Jackson, DC. Brown, LE. & Gowans, EJ. (2003). *Immunol Cell Bio,* Vol.81, No.1, (February 2003), pp. 63-66.

Franceschini, D.; Paroli, M. Francavilla, V. Videtta, M. Morrone, S. Labbadia, G. et al. (2009). *J Clin Invest,* Vol.119, No.3, (Feuruary 2009), pp. 551-564.

Francisco, LM. Sage, PT. & Sharpe, AH. (2010). *Immunol Rev,* Vol.236, (July 2010), pp. 219-242.

Freeman, AJ.; Pan, Y. Harvey, CE. Post, JJ. Law, MG. White, PA. et al. (2003). *J Hepatol,* Vol.38, No.3, (March 2003), pp. 349-356.

Golden-Mason, L.; Palmer, B, Klarquist, J, Mengshol, JA, Castelblanco, N, & Rosen, HR. (2007). *J Virol,* Vol.81, Vol.17, (June 2007), pp. 9249-9258.

Golden-Mason, L.; Klarquist, J. Wahed, AS. & Rosen, HR. (2008). *J Immunol,* Vol.180, No.6, (March 2008), pp. 3637-3641.

Golden-Mason, L.; Palmer, BE. Kassam, N. Townshend-Bulson, L. Livingston, S. McMahon, BJ. et al. (2009). *J Virol,* Vol.83, No.18, (July 2009), pp. 9122-9130.

Gowans, EJ.; Roberts, S. Jones, K. Dinatale, I. Latour, PA. Chua, B. et al. (2010). *J Hepatol,* Vol.53, No.4, (June 2010), pp. 599-607.

Guidotti, LG; Ishikawa, T. Hobbs, MV. Matzke, B. Schreiber, R. & Chisari, FV. (1996). *Immunity,* Vol.4, No.1, (January 1996), pp. 25-36.

Guidotti, LG; Rochford, R. Chung, J. Shapiro, M. Purcell, R. & Chisari, FV. (1999). *Science,* Vol.284, No.5415, (April 1999), pp. 825-829.

Guidotti, LG. & Chisari, FV. (2001).. *Annu Rev Immunol,* Vol.19, pp. 65-91.

Ha, SJ.; West, EE. Araki, K. Smith, KA. & Ahmed, R. (2008). *Immunol Rev,* Vol.223, (June 2008), pp. 317-333.

Heathcote, J.; McHutchison, J. Lee, S. Tong, M. Benner, K. Minuk, G. et al. (1999). *Hepatology,* Vol.30, No.2, (August 1999), pp. 531-536.

Helvaci, M.; Kizilgunesler, A. Kasirga, E. Ozbal, E. Kuzu, M. & Sozen, G. (2004). *J Gastroenterol Hepatol,* Vol.19, No.7, (July 2004), pp. 785-791.

Hong, Y.; Peng, Y. Mi, M. Munn, DH. Wang, GQ. & He ,Y. (2011). *Vaccine,* (Mar 2011)

Iino, S.; Toyota, J. Kumada, H. Kiyosawa, K. Kakumu, S. Sata, M. et al. (2005). *J Viral Hepat,* Vol.12, No.3, (May 2005), pp. 300-306.

Jiang, WZ.; Fan, Y. Liu, X. Zhang, YL. Wen, JJ. Hao, WL. et al. (2008). *Antiviral Res,* Vol.77, No.1, (September 2007), pp. 50-55.

Ju, Y.; Hou, N. Zhang, XN., Zhao, D. Liu, Y. Wang, JJ. et al. (2009). *Cell Mol Immunol,* Vol.6, No.1, (February 2009), pp.35-43.

Kakimi, K.; Guidotti. LG, Koezuka. Y & Chisari, FV. (2000). *J Exp Med,* Vol.192, No.7, (October 2000), pp. 921-930.

Kakimi, K; Lane, TE. Wieland, S. Asensio, VC. Campbell, IL. Chisari, FV. et al. (2001). *J Exp Med,* Vol.194, No.12, (December 2001), pp. 1755-1766.

Kimura, K.; Kakimi, K. Wieland, S. Guidotti, LG. & Chisari, FV. (2002a). *J Immunol,* Vol.169, No.9, (November 2002), pp. 5188-5195.

Kimura, K.; Kakimi, K. Wieland, S. Guidotti, LG. Chisari FV. (2002b) *J Virol,* Vol.76, No.21, (November 2002), pp. 10702-10707.

Klade, CS.; Wedemeyer, H. Berg T. Hinrichsen, H. Cholewinska, G. Zeuzem, S. et al. (2008). *Gastroenterology,* Vol.134, No.5, (March 2008), pp. 1385-1395.

Klein A, Hemed N, Segol O, Thalenfeld B, Engelhardt D, Rabbani E, et al. (2003). *Am J Gastroenterol,* Vol.98, No.11, (November 2003), pp. 2505-2515.

Koziel, MJ.; Dudley, D. Afdhal, N. Grakoui, A. Rice, CM. Choo, QL. et al. (1995). *J Clin Invest,* Vol.96, No.5, (November 1995), pp. 2311-2321.

Lechner, F.; Wong, DK. Dunbar, PR. Chapman, R. Chung, RT. Dohrenwend, P. et al. (2000). *J Exp Med.* Vol.191, No9, (May 2000), pp. 1499-1512.

Lee, HW.; Lee, JI. Um, SH. Ahn, SH. Chang, HY. Park, YK. et al. (2008). *J Gastroenterol Hepatol,* Vol.23, No.5, (May 2008), pp. 729-735.

Li, J.; Wu, W. Peng, G. Chen, F. Bai, M. Zheng, M. et al. (2010). *Immunol Cell Biol,* Vol.88, No.8, (May 2010), pp. 834-841.

Luo, J.; Li J. Chen, RL. Nie, L. Huang, J. Liu, ZW. et al. (2010). *Vaccine,* Vol.28, No.13, (January 2010), pp. 2497-2504.

Maini, MK.; Boni, C. Lee, CK. Larrubia, JR. Reignat, S. Ogg, GS. et al. (2000). *J Exp Med,* Vol.191, No.8, (April 2000), pp. 1269-1280.

Mancini-Bourgine, M.; Fontaine, H. Scott-Algara, D. Pol, S. Bréchot, C. & Michel, ML. (2004). *Hepatology,* Vol.40, No.4, (October 2004), pp. 874-882.

Mancini-Bourgine, M.; Fontaine, H., Bréchot, C. Pol, S. & Michel, ML. (2006). *Vaccine,* Vol.24, No.21, (August 2005), pp. 4482-4489.

Martin, J.; Bosch, O. Moraleda, G. Bartolome, J. Quiroga, JA. & Carreño, V. (1993). *Hepatology,* Vol.18, No.4, (October 1993), pp. 775-780.

Martin-Blondel, G.; Gales, A. Bernad, J. Cuzin, L. Delobel, P. Barange, K. et al. (2009). *J Viral Hepat,* Vol.16, No.7, (March 2009), pp. 485-491.

McMahan, RH.; Golden-Mason, L. Nishimura, MI. McMahon, BJ. Kemper, M. Allen, TM. et al. (2010). *J Clin Invest,* Vol.120, No.12, (November 2010), pp. 4546-4557.

Menne, S.; Tennant, BC. Gerin, JL. & Cote, PJ. *J Virol,* Vol.81, No.19, (July 2007), pp. 10614-10624.

Miller, DS.; Boyle, D. Feng, F. Reaiche, GY. Kotlarski, I. Colonno, R. et al. (2008). *Virology,* Vol.373, No.2, (April 2008), pp. 329-341.

Miyara, M. & Sakaguchi, S. (2011). *Immunol Cell Biol,* Vol.89, No.3, (February 2011), pp. 346-351.

Nakamoto, N.; Cho, H. Shaked, A. Olthoff, K. Valiga, ME. Kaminski, M. et al. *PLoS Pathog,* Vol.5, No.2, (February 2009), e1000313.

Nan, XP.; Zhang, Y. Yu, HT. Li, Y. Sun, RL. Wang, JP. et al. (2010). *Viral Immunol,* Vol.23, No.1, (February 2010), pp. 63-70.

Op den Brouw, ML.; Binda, RS. van Roosmalen, MH. Protzer, U. Janssen, HL. van der Molen, RG. et al. (2009). *Immunology,* Vol.126, No.2, (June 2008), pp. 280-289.

Peng, G.; Luo, B. Li, J. Zhao, D. Wu, W. Chen, F. et al. (2011). *J Clin Immunol,* Vol.31, No.2, (April 2011), pp. 195-204.

Penna, A.; Pilli, M. Zerbini, A. Orlandini, A. Mezzadri, S. Sacchelli, L. et al. (2007). *Hepatology,* Vol.45, No.3, (Mar 2007), pp. 588-601.

Pol, S.; Nalpa,s B. Driss, F. Michel, ML. Tiollais, P. Denis, J. et al. (2001). *J Hepatol,* Vol.34, No.6, (June 2001), pp. 917-921.

Poo, JL.; Sánchez Avila, F. Kershenobich, D. García Samper, X. Torress-Ibarra, R. Góngora, J. et al. (2008). *Ann Hepatol,* Vol.7, No.4, (October-December 2008), pp.369-375.

Raziorrouh, B.; Schraut, W. Gerlach, T. Nowack, D. Grüner, NH. Ulsenheimer, A. et al. (2010). *Hepatology,* Vol.52, No.6, (Novemver 2010), pp. 1934-1947.

Rehermann, B. *Baillieres Clin Gastroenterol.* (1996).Vol.10, No. 3 (September 1996), pp. 483-500.

Rigopoulou, EI.; Suri, D. Chokshi, S. Mullerova, I. Rice, S. Tedder, RS. et al. (2005). *Hepatology,* Vol.42, No.5, (November 2005), pp. 1028-1036.

Rowan, AG.; Fletcher, JM. Ryan, EJ. Moran, B. Hegarty, JE. O'Farrelly, C. et al. (2008). *J Immunol,* Vol.181, No.7, (October 2008), pp. 4485-4494.

Sabat, R.; Grütz, G. Warszawska, K. Kirsch, S. Witte, E. Wolk, K. et al. (2010). *Cytokine Growth Factor Rev,* Vol.21, No.5, (Novermber 2010), pp. 331-344.

Safadi, R.; Israeli, E. Papo, O. Shibolet, O. Melhem, A. Bloch, A. et al. (2003). *Am J Gastroenterol,* Vol.98, No.11, (November 2003), pp. 2505-2515.

Semmo, N. & Klenerman, P. (2007). *World J Gastroenterol.* Vol.13, No.36, (September 2007), pp. 4831-4838.

Senturk, H.; Tabak, F. Ozaras, R. Erdem, L. Canbakan, B. Mert, A. et al. (2009). *Dig Dis Sci,* Vol.54, No.9, (November 2008), pp. 2026-2030.

Shimizu, Y.; Guidotti, LG., Fowler, P. & Chisari, FV. (1998). *J Immunol,* Vol.161, No.9, (November 1998), pp. 4520-4529.

Shoukry, NH.; Sidney, J. Sette, A. & Walker, CM. (2004). *J Immunol,* Vol.172, No.1, (January 2004), pp. 483-92.

Stoop JN, Claassen MA, Woltman AM, Binda RS, Kuipers EJ, Janssen HL, et al. (2008). Clin Immunol. Vol.129, No.3, (December 2008), pp. 419-427.

Sturm, N.; Thélu, MA. Camous, X. Dimitrov, G. Ramzan, M. Dufeu-Duchesne, T. et al. (2010). *J Hepatol,* Vol.53, No.1, (April 2010), pp. 25-35.

Szkaradkiewicz, A.; Jopek, A. & Wysocki, J. (2005). *Antiviral Res,* Vol.66, No.1, (April 2005), pp. 23-27.

Takaki, A.; Tatsukawa, M. Iwasaki, Y. Koike, K. Noguchi, Y. Shiraha, H. et al. (2009). *J Viral Hepat,* Vol.17, No.8, (October 2009), pp. 555-562.

Thermet, A.; Buronfosse, T. Werle-Lapostolle, B. Chevallier, M. Pradat, P. Trepo, C. (2008). *J Gen Virol,* Vol.89, Vol. Pt 5, (May 2008), pp. 1192-1201.

Tsai, SL.; Liaw, YF. Chen, MH. Huang, CY.& Kuo, GC. (1997). Detection of type 2-like T-helper cells in hepatitis C virus infection: implications for hepatitis C virus chronicity. *Hepatology,* Vol.25, No.2, (February 1997), pp 449-458.

Urbani, S.; Amadei, B. Tola, D. Pedrazzi, G. Sacchelli, L. Cavallo, MC. et al. (2008). *J Hepatol,* Vol.48, No.4, (January 2008), pp. 548-558.

Vandepapelière, P.; Lau, GK. Leroux-Roels, G. Horsmans, Y. Gane, E. Tawandee, T. et al. (2007). *Vaccine,* Vol.25, No.51, (October 2007), pp. 8585-8597.

Wang, FS.; Xing, LH. Liu, MX. Zhu, CL. Liu, HG. Wang, HF. et al. (2001). *World J Gastroenterol,* Vol.7, No.4, (August 2001), pp537-541.

Wang, J.; Zhu, Q., Zhang, T. & Yu, H. (2002). *Chin Med J,* Vol.115, No.12, (December 2002), pp. 1824-1828.

Wang, S.; Han, Q. Zhang, N. Chen, J., Liu, Z. Zhang, G. et al. (2010). *Immunol Lett,* Vol.127, No.2, (October 2009), pp. 143-149.

Webster, GJ.; Reignat, S., Maini, MK. Whalley, SA. Ogg, GS. King, A. et al. (2000). *Hepatology,* Vol.32, No.5, (November 2000), pp. 1117-1124.

Webster, GJ. & Bertoletti, A. (2001). *Mol Immunol,* Vol.38, No.6, (December 2001), pp. 467-473.

Woltman, AM.; Ter Borg, MJ. Binda, RS. Sprengers, D. von Blomberg, BM. Scheper, RJ. et al. (2009). *Antivir Ther,* Vol.14, No.6, (2009), pp. 809-818.

Xing, Y.; Huang, Z. Lin, Y. Yang, Z. Yao, X. Guo, S. et al. (2008). *Vaccine,* Vol.26, No.40, (April 2008), pp. 5145-5152.

Xu D, Fu J, Jin L, Zhang H, Zhou C, Zou Z, et al. (2006). *J Immunol,* Vol.177, No.1, (July 2006), pp. 739-747.

Yao, ZQ.; King, E., Prayther, D. Yin, D. & Moorman, J. (2007). *Viral Immunol,* Vol.20. No.2, (Summer 2007), pp. 276-287.

You, J.; Zhuang, L. Cheng, HY. Yan, SM. Yu, L. Huang, JH.et al. (2006). *World J Gastroenterol,* Vol.12, No.41, (November 2006), pp. 6715-6721.

Yutani, S.; Komatsu, N. Shichijo, S. Yoshida, K. Takedatsu, H. Itou, M. et al. (2009). *Cancer Sci,* Vol.100, No.10, (June 2009), pp. 1935-1942.

Zeuzem, S. & Carreño, V. (2001). *Antiviral Res,* Vol.52, No.2, (November 2001), pp. 181-188.

Zhang, Y.; Liu, Y. Moxley, KM. Golden-Mason, L. Hughes, MG. & Liu, T. (2010). *PLoS Pathog,* Vol.6, No.7, (July 2010), e1001018.

Zhang, YY.; Chen, EQ. Yang, J. Duan, YR. & Tang, H. (2009). *Virol J,* Vol.25, No.6, (May 2009), pp.63.

4

Evolution of Viral Hepatitis: Role of Psychosocial Stress

Cristin Constantin Vere, Costin Teodor Streba, Ion Rogoveanu, Alin Gabriel Ionescu and Letitia Adela Maria Streba
University of Medicine and Pharmacy of Craiova
Romania

1. Introduction

Psychological stress, as defined by modern science, appears when an individual balances existing threats, being real or imaginary, and after confronting them with his or hers current resources, and finds the later to be inadequate. In practice, this occurs when experiences are judged to be exceeding adaptive capacities by an individual, therefore over-soliciting the mental defense mechanisms and coping capabilities. The above definition and context excludes psychiatric disorders that may impair the integration capacities of an individual. In the following chapter, psychiatric disorders resulting from stressful events are also excluded.
Chronic psychosocial stress is possibly the most complex and powerful harming agent, as its repetitive nature enables it to constantly follow a patient during the onset and the course of chronic disease.
The idea that stressful events in a life of a person can influence his or hers response to illness is an idea that appeared from ancient times, despite a lack of scientific evidence. However, recent advances in the field of psychoneuroimmunology led to a new perspective on the issue. The scientific community devoted its attention to designing experiments and studies in order to document the effects and interactions between psychological and physical stress, and the well-being of a living organism.
Within the last two decades, several studies revealed new interactions between endocrine response systems, such as the hypothalamic-pituitary-adrenal axis (HPA) or the sympathetic-adrenal-medullary (SAM) system, and various pathologies. Moreover, it has been proven that the central nervous system and especially the autonomous component exert regulatory effects on the immunity of the organism. The two regulatory bodies are deeply interconnected, numerous links at various levels critically determining the end function and outcome of the immune response.
Liver disease was demonstrated to be heavily influenced by perceived chronic stress during several human and animal studies. The effects of chronic viral hepatitis on liver parenchyma are well known, however the idea that real-life events, independent from the disease itself, can influence the course of this disease, is relatively new.

2. Historical background

From ancient times, the idea of the mind-body union has been deeply rooted into human beliefs. Religion as well as empiric medicine documented the relationship between the state of mind and the organic well-being of an individual. Hippocrates (460-377 BC) identified a link between negative emotions and incidents and somatic disorders, introducing the concept of psychosomatics. Socrates (469-399 BC) proclaimed as well that in order to cure an individual, the physician should take into account the physical illness or defect, as well as the spiritual, or as we would call it in modern times, the psychic component. Galen (AD 129-199) further implemented the concept of negative emotions, such as anger, discontent or grief, as being "diseases".

However, this conceptual unity was contested during later years, the dispute being irrevocably solved by Rene Descartes (1596-1650) who proposed that the body is simply a machine that obeys the laws of physics, while the soul, which he placed in the pineal gland, was completely separated, and governed the mind of an individual. For the following 300 years all philosophical and medical writings approached the mind-body dichotomy from the same perspective.

Early twentieth century experiments, pioneered by Ivan Pavlov, William Beaumont and Steward Wolf, began to elucidate the relationship between the nervous system and different organs and their respective pathologies.

The last three decades of scientific research were crucial in the understanding of the intricate relationships between the

3. The anatomical foundation and the mechanisms of the organic response to stress

3.1 The central stress mechanism

Currently, it is widely acknowledged that a central stress mechanism exists, composed of different brain structures such as the lateral prefrontal cortex and the medial prefrontal structures, which in turn are connected with the amygdala and the paraventricular nucleus of the hypothalamus.

Output from these structures is projected onto the pontomedullary nuclei and the pituitary gland. The signals from this central system are conveyed to the sympathetic nervous system components regulated through autonomic neurotransmitters (epinephrine and norepinephrine). (Glaser R, 2005;)

The neuroendocrine component is represented by the functional axis composed from the hypothalamus, the pituitary and the adrenal glands (the HPA axis), regulated through circulating glucocorticoids. (Chrousos GP, 1992; Kemeny ME and Schedlowski M, 2007)

Pituitary hormones (prolactine and growth hormone) are released along with the adrenocorticotropic hormone (ACTH), neuropeptide Y (NPY) and opioids are actively released during stressful events. They directly influence antibody as well as cellular mediated immune response. ((Malarkey and Mills, 2007; Blalock and Smith, 2007)

All structures of the immune system receive sympathetic noradrenergic innervation, while B and T cellular lines express beta and alpha adrenoreceptors. (Kelley et al., 2007) The production and release of various cytokines and the circulation of leukocytes are also influenced by adrenaline and noradrenaline, neuromediators which are increasingly secreted during stress response. This increased sympathetic response stimulates the functions of the next major component in the stress response mechanism, the HPA axis, which in turn secretes elevated quantities of glucocorticoids, thus impairing the immune response. (Glaser and Kiecolt-Glaser, 2005)

3.2 The hypothalamic-pituitary-adrenal axis, glucocorticoids and the sympathetic nervous system

The HPA axis represents, as stated above, the functional and anatomical system that regulates glucocorticoid secretion, playing a major role in the adaptive response of a normally-functioning organism. It is under direct neural control, receiving sympathetic innervation through short and long feedback circuits from the hypothalamus and other central structures.

Hence, it is deeply interconnected with the systemic and sympathetic adrenomedullary systems, both key components of the stress system, collaborating for the maintenance of basal homeostasis. The corticotrophin-releasing hormone (CRH) and noradrenergic neurons of the central stress system are in close relation through a two-way feedback mechanism (Sanders VM and Kavelaars A, 2007) that assures inter-regulated levels of production of norepinephrine and CRH. (Sawchenko PE et al, 1993)

The hypothalamus represents the main regulatory structure of the HPA axis. It balances glucocorticoid secretion through the release of CRH and arginine vasopressin (AVP), with proinflammatory effects. These mediators are released in inflammation areas, while plasmatic concentrations remain low, thus proving their local effect in the inflammatory process. (Karalis K et al, 1991) The hypothalamic activity is up-regulated by the serotoninergic and cholinergic systems, and its activity is inhibited by the opioid-peptide and the gamma-aminobutiric acid-benzodiazepine systems existing at cerebral level. Substance P stimulates the central noradrenergic system, while inhibiting hypothalamic CRH-secreting neurons. (Culman J et al, 1993; Larsen PJ et al, 1993; Jessop DS et al, 1992)

Hormones secreted by the adrenal medulla, such as corticotrophin, are the most important factors that regulate the secretion of glucocorticoids by the HPA. (Hinson JP. 1990; Calogero AE et al, 1992)

Secreted glucocorticoids regulate T-helper-1 and 2 responses to viral infection by inhibiting the production of Interleukin 12 (IL-12) and Tumor Necrosis Factor Alpha (TNF Alpha). Several other interleukines (IL), such as IL-2 and cytokines IL-10 and IL-4 are stimulated through their actions. All these exert a pro-inflammatory role and occur under the influence of stress-related mechanisms. (Glaser and Kiecolt-Glaser, 2005).

Glucocorticoids also cause resistance to cytokines and stimulate eosinophil apoptosis, inhibit adhesion molecules and their specific receptors expressions (Cronstein BN et al, 1992) and exacerbate the acute phase reaction (Hirano T et al, 1990). Pituitary hormones such as corticotrophin and especially beta-endorphin increase the immune response level and facilitate local inflammatory activity, (Bateman A et al, 1989) along with having analgesic effects (Schafer M et al, 1994).

3.3 The HPA axis role in acute and chronic liver inflammation

As already stated above, the activation of the HPA axis represents a key element of the normal response to stressor factors. The end result of this stimulation is the active secretion of glucocorticoids from the adrenal cortex, which is a natural process designed to improve survival chances in a fight-or-run scenario, usually associated with the notion of "exterior stress". This process, however, is involved in the control of the inflammatory response, which, in turn, can also interact by stimulation of the vagal afferents and thus activation of the HPA axis.

Patients with chronic liver diseases, such as viral hepatitis, express delayed cortisol clearance and altered cortisol binding at plasma level. Elevated plasma cytokine levels are common in chronic inflammatory diseases, and chronic exposure to high levels of circulating cytokines is associated with HPA axis failure or dysfunction. (Turnbull AV and Rivier CL, 1999)

Experimental data suggest that chronic liver injury results in elevated TNF-alpha and IL-6 levels, as well as more specific cellular alterations at hypothalamic level, such as mRNA depletion and impaired protein expression resulting in decreased levels of secreted CRH, which in turn impairs the activation of HPA axis mechanisms. (Swain MG et al, 1993) Thus, lower levels of circulating hormones, consecutive to the independent action of an exterior stressor, may be a promoter of hepatic inflammation, concomitant to the usual viral effects.

Acute inflammatory injury of the liver in a rodent model resulted in the rapid activation of the HPA axis, with consecutive rises in circulating glucocorticoid (GC) levels. When the physiological effects of GCs are inhibited, the inflammatory response is enhanced, resulting in an increase mortality rate. (Swain MG et al, 1999) This in turn can be prevented by the administration of exogenous GCs. (Swain MG, 2000) The protective effect of GCs can partially be attributed to the fact that they mediate the synthesis and release of IL-10 at hepatic level, specifically by the liver-specific macrophage system, the Kupffer cells. They also produce a number of inflammatory mediators, such as IL-1, IL-6, TNF-alpha and the nitric oxide (NO), all of them up-regulated during liver inflammation. These effects are attributed to indirect mechanisms, as they interfere with the production of proinflammatory transcription factors such as (NF)-kB and the activator protein AP-1, or to direct mechanisms which operate at the level of mRNA stability and gene transcription.

Liao et al (Liao et al, 1995) studied the effects of corticosterone, at both normal and stress levels, on an isolated perfused rat liver. He observed that the GC increased the release of TNF-alpha and IL-6. Later studies provided evidence that psychological stress itself can have the exact effect, possibly by following the same pathways. (Tjandra K et al, 2001) The hepatic levels of inflammatory cytokines and compounds are differently influenced by GCs, as TNF-alpha seems to be the first to be altered, followed by IL 1 and IL 6.

The hepatitis C virus was directly linked to the recruitment of cellular effectors implicated in liver inflammation, during viral disease. Chemokines, being important mediators of liver inflammation, experience an increased expression during HCV infection. As dexamethasone, synthetic GC is routinely used in pretreatment phases, and was shown to attenuate endotoxins and cytokine expression of chemokines in immune cells during liver inflammation, we can suggest a theoretical link between stress-levels of endogenous GCs and chemokine levels during viral hepatitis.

Another critical component of the immune system is represented by T cells. In the liver, they are actively involved in the initiation, propagation and maintenance of the inflammatory disease. GCs were proven to specifically interact with T-cell proliferation in the liver, adrenal steroids being regulators of the T helper (Th) lymphocyte cytokine secretion. Many hormones that circulate in plasma as inactive forms are transformed into their active forms within the liver. Activation of the HPA axis under stress impairs the release of Th1 cytokines, thus shifting the profile towards Th2 dominance, as documented by Iwakabe et al (Iwakabe K et al, 1998) in a restrain-stress study on a rodent model.

Circulating GCs induce T cell apoptosis. During the course of viral hepatitis, increased GCs levels at a hepatic level, following HPA activation, correlate with lower levels of activated T-cells at the same level.

Tamada et al (Tamada K et al, 1998) proved that administration of dexamethasone increases production of IL-4 hepatic natural killer (NK) 1.11-positive T cells, demonstrating that this cellular line is resistant to apoptosis induced by GCs. This study comes to support the theory that HPA may actively regulate the Th1/Th2 balance during acute or chronic stress exposure.

Proliferation of liver natural killer T (NKT) cells and the up-regulation of the Fas antigen on hepatocytes follow the increased GC production by the HPA axis. This conclusion is supported by research conducted by Chida and his team (Chida Y et al, 2004; Chida Y et al, 2006), who induced physical and psychological stress to rats by inescapable foot-shock.

Restrain stress, another standardized method of assessing psychophysical stress in animal studies, was found to increase the proportion of NK cells in the mouse liver through increased HPA activity and higher than normal GC concentrations. (Shimizu et al, 2000)

Recent studies shown that monocyte chemotactic protein (MCP 1) and macrophage inflammatory protein (MIP 2) distribute NK cells along with other chemokines, thus suggesting that GCs may influence this sub-population through down-regulation of these substances (Kawakami K et al, 2001; Faunce DE et al, 2000)

Neutrophils are important in the early phases of hepatic inflammation. Circulating GCs have an inhibitory effect on neutrophil recruitment, as they down-regulate the expression of adhesion molecules, thus impairing chemotaxis.

3.4 The parasympathetic nervous system and hepatic inflammation

Recently, the main component of the parasympathetic feedback loop-mechanism that regulates liver inflammation was identified to be the "cholinergic anti-inflammatory pathway", this theory stating that efferent nerve fibers exist, supplementing the normal afferent pathways that sent information to the central nervous system from the hepatic site. Several cytokines such as IL-1 beta and TNF alpha seem to be implicated in the transduction process. In an in vivo macrophage culture, efferent vagus nerve was found to inhibit TNF alpha by releasing acetylcholine, when stimulated by endotoxins. This effect was proven to be dependent to nicotine acetylcholine receptor alpha 7 subunit (Borovikova LV et al, 2000; Wang H et al, 2003; Chida et al, 2006).

Several studies on transplanted and denervated livers show that inflammatory and immune components are severely impaired by the lack of sympathetic and parasympathetic innervations.

Growing evidence that anti-stress therapies known in traditional and standard medicine seem to stimulate the vagal influence on the liver, thus decreasing the immune response. (Zachariae R et al, 2001; Lux G et al, 1994)

4. The influence of psychosocial stress on viral hepatitis

Not many clinical studies evaluate the relationship between viral hepatitis B or C and stress response in a real-life setting. A number of studies did however underline the different mechanisms between the primary anatomical and functional systems in the human body and the intrinsic mechanisms regulating hepatic inflammation, the main morphological change encountered during the course of viral liver infection.

Nagano et al (Nagano J et al, 2004) indicated in a clinical trial that a possible correlation exists between psychosocial stress and the severity of chronic hepatitis C. His team assessed levels of perceived stressor events through standardized stress questionnaires specifically designed to also provide information regarding personality types. Type 1 personality subjects are prone to disease due to the nature of their personal traits, being likely to be affected throughout chronic stress. Both type 1 personality traits as well as psychosocial stress positively correlated with the severity of chronic hepatitis C. Stress levels were assessed using items from the Grossarth-Maticek theory, which states that type-1 personality subjects are prone to developing chronic diseases. The severity of chronic hepatitis C was assessed through the levels of ALAT, platelet counts, albumin and total bilirubin levels, resulting two hepatitis groups and one cirrhosis group, containing those patients that exhibited signs of this pathology. Platelet count and serum albumin levels were positively correlated with levels of stress, and also proved to be good assessors for the severity of chronic hepatitis. ASAT values were strongly correlated with stress levels and type 1 personality types, thus establishing a connection between stress and the severity of chronic hepatitis C.

A link between chronic hepatitis B and depression scores and psychosocial stressors were assessed in a group of 50 HbsAg-positive Korean immigrants. (Kunkel et al, 2000). Depression scores, psychosocial factors and social support were evaluated and compared with biological markers of liver dysfunction, including hepatic transaminases, albumin levels and prothrombin times. These routine clinic follow-up values were correlated with scores obtained from short form Beck Depression Inventory questionnaires. Higher scores were significantly associated with elevated levels of transaminases; however albumin and PT levels did not correlate with stress scores.

Psychological implications of hepatitis C virus diagnosis were evaluated by a number of studies. Muzaffar et al (Muzaffar L et al, 2005) proved that the diagnosis of HCV is considered more stressful than divorce or material loss or house relocation. His study of 98 patients infected with hepatitis C and 100 controls compared stress and anxiety levels regarding the diagnosis of HCV with other life-changing events including death of a close relative, loss of marital or material status or move to another city.

A study performed by Laurent Castera (Castera L et al, 2006) concluded that the psychological impact of chronic hepatitis C and emotional burden of such diagnoses are considerable, even when liver disease is insignificant.

5. Psychosocial stress and vaccination against hepatitis B

Hepatitis B currently represents a major health burden in many areas around the globe. The possibility of an effective vaccination is vital for controlling the effects hepatitis B viruses may have on exposed populations. Current studies estimate that a proportion of over 90% of the healthy subjects respond well to vaccination; however, the remaining 10% may not possess protective antibody titers at the end of the vaccination period. (Zajac BA et al, 1986)

Chronic environmental stress exposure is common in several social settings, such as academic mediums which require extensive examination periods, unfulfilled marriages or job-related distress. These situations were shown to have a negative impact on all components of the immune response. This relationship can best be described by studying the effects stressors have on vaccination outcome, as this procedure clearly reflects the efficiency of the innate immune system against disease.

Clinical studies which take into account stress exposure when assessing vaccination protection against hepatitis B are especially useful both for quantifying the effects of psychological stress on the immune response, and naturally for determining the optimum clinical settings for a successful vaccination campaign.

Burns et al (Burns VE et al, 2002) evaluated the stress and coping level of 265 first-year medical school undergraduates who completed the standard three-dose recombinant hepatitis B vaccination program. Test questionnaires were given to the participants, assessing life events of the past 12 months as well as coping types through the brief cope questionnaire and a short survey on individual health behaviors. Then their serum antibody levels were determined quantitatively. They found significant relations between stress questionnaire scores and antibody titers, while determining that coping and acceptance coping are significant predictors for antibody status. Life events exposure, sleep duration and physical exercises also proved to significantly improve antibody status post-vaccination.

Another study (Marsland AL et al, 2006) examined 84 graduate students who received standard hepatitis B vaccination series. Subjects underwent a battery of questionnaires, and blood samples were evaluated. Their results showed that higher scores, measuring a positive dispositional affect (thus a sense of well-being and fulfillment), positively correlated with greater antibody response to hepatitis B vaccination. Physical activity also proved to provide a protective role.

The general consensus of these studies is that further studies should overcome obvious limitations such as retrospective design or small cohorts, and that experimental models can be devised in order to assess antibody status after hepatitis B vaccination.

6. Conclusion

Current evidence proves a definite link between psychosocial stress levels and the status of liver hepatitis. The effects on the immune response ultimately lead to an exacerbation of the inflammatory response at hepatic level.

Recent advances were made in understanding the complete interactions between stress, neuroimmunomodulation and ultimately the onset and progress of viral infections.

Clinical implications are profound, as translational studies deciphering intrinsic cellular mechanisms and pathways lead the way to a better understanding of viral liver infection, thus improving the standard of care in this pathology.

Further studies are needed in order to fully understand the complex interactions between the social environment and chronic viral hepatitis.

7. References

Bateman A, Singh A, Kral T, Solomon S. The immunehypothalamic-pituitary-adrenal axis. Endocr Rev 1989; 10:92-112.

Borovikova LV, Ivanva S, Zhang M et al. Vagus nerve stimulation attenuates the systemic inflammatory response to endotoxin. Nature 2000; 405: 458–62.

Blalock, J.E., Smith, E.M., 2007. Conceptual development of the immune system as a sixth sense. Brain Behav. Immun. 21, 23–33.

Burns VE, Carroll D, Ring C, Harrison LK, Drayson M. Stress, coping, and hepatitis B antibody status. Psychosom Med 2002; 64: 287-293

Calogero AE, Norton JA, Sheppard BC, Listwak SJ, Cromack DT, Wall R, Jensen RT, Chrousos GP. Pulsatile activation of the hypothalamic-pituitary-adrenal axis during major surgery. Metabolism 1992; 41: 839-845.

Castera L, Constant A, Bernard PH, de Ledinghen V, Couzigou P. Psychological impact of chronic hepatitis C: Comparison with other stressful life events and chronic diseases. World J Gastroenterol 2006; 12(10): 1545-1550

Chida Y, Sudo N, Sonoda J, Sogawa H, Kubo C. Electric foot shock stress-induced exacerbation of alpha-galactosylceramide-triggered apoptosis in mouse liver. Hepatology 2004; 39: 1131-1140

Chida Y, Sudo N, Kubo C. Does stress exacerbate liver diseases? J Gastroenterol Hepatol 2006; 21: 202-208

Chrousos GP. Regulation and dysregulation of the hypothalamic-pituitary-adrenal axis. The corticotropinreleasing hormone perspective. Endocrinol Metab Clin North Am 1992; 21: 833-858

Cronstein BN, Kimmel SC, Levin RI, Martiniuk F, Weissmann G. A mechanism for the antiinflammatory effects

Culman J, Tschope C, Jost N, Itoi K, Unger T. Substance P and neurokinin A induced desensitization to cardiovascular and behavioral effects: evidence for the involvement of different tachykinin receptors. Brain Res 1993; 625: 75-83.

Faunce DE, Sonoda KH, Streilein JS. MIP-2 recruits NKT cells to the spleen during tolerance induction. J. Immunol. 2001; 166: 313–21.

Glaser, R., 2005. Stress-associated immune dysregulation and its importance for human health: a personal history of psychoneuroimmunology. Brain Behav. Immun. 17, 321–328.

Glaser, R., Kiecolt-Glaser, J.K., 2005. Stress-induced immune dysfunction: implications for health. Nat. Rev. Immunol. 5, 243–251.

Hinson JP. Paracrine control of adrenocortical function: a new role for the medulla? J Endocrinol 1990; 124: 7-9.

Hirano T, Akira S, Taga T, Kishimoto T. Biological and clinical aspects of interleukin 6. Immunol Today 1990; 11: 443-449.

Iwakabe K, Shimada M, Ohta A, Yahata T, Ohmi Y, Habu S, and Nishimura T. The restraint stress drives a shift in Th1/Th2 balance toward Th2-dominant immunity in mice. Immunol Lett 62: 39–43, 1998.

Jessop DS, Chowdrey HS, Larsen PJ, Lightman SL. Substance P: multifunctional peptide in the hypothalamopituitary system? J Endocrinol 1992; 132: 331-337.

Kawakami K, Kinjo Y, Uezu K et al. Monocyte chemoattractant protein-1-dependent increase of V alpha 14 NKT cells in lungs and their roles in Th1 response and host defense in Cryptococcal infection. J. Immunol. 2001; 167: 6525–32.

Karalis K, Sano H, Redwine J, Listwak S, Wilder RL, Chrousos GP. Autocrine or paracrine inflammatory actions

Kelley, K.W., Weigent, D.A., Kooijman, R., 2007. Protein hormones and immunity. Brain Behav. Immun. 21, 384–392.

Kemeny ME, Schedlowski M. Understanding the interaction between psychosocial stress and immune-related diseases: A stepwise progression. Brain, Behavior, and Immunity 21 (2007) 1009–1018.

Kunkel EJ, Kim JS, Hann HW, Oyesanmi O, Menefee LA, Field HL, Lartey PL, Myers RE. Depression in Korean immigrants with hepatitis B and related liver diseases. Psychosomatics 2000; 41: 472-480.

Larsen PJ, Jessop D, Patel H, Lightman SL, Chowdrey HS. Substance P inhibits the release of anterior pituitary adrenocorticotrophin via a central mechanism involving corticotrophin-releasing factor-containing neurons in the hypothalamic paraventricular nucleus. J Neuroendocrinol 1993; 5: 99-105.

Liao J, Keiser JA, Scales WE, Kunkel SL, and Kluger MJ. Role of corticosterone in TNF and IL-6 production in isolated perfused rat liver. Am J Physiol Regulatory Integrative Comp Physiol 268: R699–R706, 1995.

Lux G, Hagel J, Backer P et al. Acupuncture inhibits vagal gastric acid secretion stimulated by sham feeding in healthy subjects. Gut 1994; 35: 1026–9.

Malarkey, W.B., Mills, P.J., 2007. Endocrinology: the active partner in PNI research. Brain Behav. Immun. 21, 161–168.

Marsland AL, Cohen S, Rabin BS, Manuck SB. Trait positive affect and antibody response to hepatitis B vaccination. Brain Behav Immun 2006; 20: 261-269

Muzaffar L Gill, Muslim Atiq, Syma Sattar And Nasir Khokhar. Psychological implications of hepatitis C virus diagnosis. Journal of Gastroenterology and Hepatology (2005) 20, 1741–1744 of corticotropin-releasing hormone in vivo. Science 1991; 254: 421-423.

Nagano J, Nagase S, Sudo N, Kubo C. Psychosocial stress, personality, and the severity of chronic hepatitis C.

Psychosomatics 2004; 45: 100-106

Sanders, V.M., Kavelaars, A., 2007. Adrenergic regulation of immunity. In: Ader, R., Felten, D.L., Cohen, N. (Eds.), Psychoneuroimmunology. Academic Press, New York.

Sawchenko PE, Imaki T, Potter E, Kovacs K, Imaki J, Vale W. The functional neuroanatomy of corticotropin-releasing factor. Ciba Found Symp 1993; 172: 5-21.

Schafer M, Carter L, Stein C. Interleukin 1 beta and corticotropin-releasing factor inhibit pain by releasing opioids from immune cells in inflamed tissue. Proc Natl Acad Sci U S A. 1994 May 10;91(10):4219-23.

Shimizu T, Kawamura T, Miyaji C et al. Resistance of extrathymic T cells to stress and the role of endogenous glucocorticoids in stress associated immunosuppression. Scand. J. Immunol. 2000; 51: 285–92.

Swain MG, Patchev V, Vergalla J, Chrousos GP, and Jones EA. Suppression of hypothalamic-pituitary-adrenal axis responsiveness to stress in a rat model of acute cholestasis. J Clin Invest 91: 1903–1908, 1993.

Swain MG, Appleyard C, Wallace J, Wong H, and Le T. Endogenous glucocorticoids released during acute toxic liver injury enhance hepatic IL-10 synthesis and release. Am J Physiol Gastrointest Liver Physiol 276: G199–G205, 1999.

Swain MG. Stress and the liver. Am J Physiol Gastrointest Liver Physiol 279:1135-1138, 2000.

Tamada K, Harada M, Abe K, Li T, Nomoto K. IL-4-producing NK1.1+ T cells are resistant to glucocorticoidinduced apoptosis: implications for the Th1/Th2 balance. J Immunol 1998; 161: 1239-1247

Tjandra K, Sharkey KA, and Swain MG. Progressive development of a Th1-type hepatic cytokine profile in rats with experimental cholangitis. Hepatology 31: 280–290, 2000.

Turnbull AV and Rivier CL. Regulation of the hypothalamicpituitary-adrenal axis by cytokines: actions and mechanisms of action. Physiol Rev 70: 1–71, 1999.

Zachariae R. Hypnosis and immunity. In: Ader R, Felten DL, Cohen N, eds. Psychoneuroimmunology, vol. 2. San Diego: Academi, 2001; 133–60.

Zajac BA, West DJ, McAleer WJ, Scolnick EM. Overview of clinical studies with hepatitis B vaccine made by recombinant DNA. J Infect 1986;13:39–45.

Wang H, Yu M, Ochani M et al. Nicotinic acetylcholine receptor a7 subunit is an essential regulator of inflammation. Nature 2003; 421: 384–8.

5

Viral Hepatitis in Solid Organ Transplant Recipients

Lisa B. VanWagner[1] and Josh Levitsky[1,2]
[1]*Department of Medicine, Division of Gastroenterology and Hepatology*
[2]*Department of Surgery, Division of Organ Transplantation at Northwestern University Feinberg School of Medicine, Chicago, Illinois*
United States of America

1. Introduction

Hepatotropic viral infections are frequent in allograft recipients and may be caused by a number of different viruses. Of these, the most important infectious agents are hepatitis B virus (HBV) and hepatitis C virus (HCV), which can cause both acute and chronic hepatitis. In addition, Hepatitis E virus (HEV), thought previously to only cause acute hepatitis in the developing world, is emerging as an increasing cause of chronic hepatitis and even cirrhosis in solid organ transplant recipients in industrialized countries(Gerolami, Moal et al. 2008; Kamar, Mansuy et al. 2008; Gerolami, Moal et al. 2009; Haagsma, Niesters et al. 2009). Hepatitis D virus (HDV) additionally plays an important role in both coinfection and superinfection of HBV in solid organ transplant recipients. In addition to the primary viral hepatitis infections, a variety of other systemic viral infections, such as the herpesviruses, cytomegalovirus (CMV), Ebstein Barr Virus (EBV), and varicella zoster virus (VZV) can have toxic effects on the liver in the posttransplant recipient. This chapter will focus primarily on the epidemiology, transmission, clinical presentation and management of the primary hepatitis viruses: HBV, HCV, HDV and HEV, following solid organ transplantation. General concepts in the prevention of post-transplant hepatotropic infections and recent advances and challenges will also be discussed.

2. Risk factors for the development of viral hepatitis post-transplant

The risk of viral hepatitis following solid organ transplant varies over time and is closely related to modifications in immunosuppression. There are three time frames, influenced by surgical factors, the level of immunosuppression, and environmental exposures, during which infections of specific types most frequently occur posttransplantation. These include the first month; the second through sixth months, and the late posttransplant period (beyond the sixth month) (Fishman 2007). With few exceptions, most viral hepatitis occurs during the middle to late periods following solid organ transplant, often due to reactivation within a recipient. However, both donor and recipient-derived infections can present in the early posttransplant period.

2.1 Epidemiologic exposures

Epidemiologic exposures, including donor-derived and recipient-derived transmission play an integral role in the timing and severity of viral hepatitis. Mandatory reporting of transplantation-associated infections has increased awareness of donor-associated infection, and all transplant centers perform some type of screening for common types of infections in order to reduce transmission from the donor to the recipient. In addition, pre-transplantation screening of recipients for common causes of viral hepatitis helps to prevent reactivation posttransplant. Finally, nosocomial transmission via blood transfusions or hemodialysis has been reported in solid-organ transplant recipients.

2.1.1 Donor-derived infections and screening recommendations

Transplanted organs can facilitate transmission of hepatitis from organ donors. Most often, these infections are latent in the transplanted tissues, however active donor infection (e.g. viremia) may also cause viral hepatitis in solid organ transplant recipients. HBV, HCV and CMV are the most commonly reported hepatotropic viruses transmitted during solid organ transplant though the incidence of transmission has decreased over the last decade due to improvements in screening and vaccination practices. Recently, HEV infection has been added as an emergent cause of chronic hepatitis in organ transplantation(Haagsma, Niesters et al. 2009).

The screening of transplant donors for infections is limited by the available technology and by the short period during which organs from deceased donors can be used. Currently, the evaluation of donors for viral hepatitis relies on an epidemiologic history for common modes of transmission (e.g. intravenous drug use) and serologic testing for antibodies to common hepatotropic viruses such as CMV, HBV (hepatitis B surface antigen (HBsAg), antibodies against hepatitis B surface antigen (anti-HBs)), HCV, EBV, and VZV. In certain situations (e.g. history of intravenous drug use or known exposure to a hepatotrophic virus) special testing using nucleic acid assays may be performed. Since seroconversion may not occur during acute infections and the sensitivity of these tests is not 100%, some active infections may remain undetected.

The 'window period' for a pathogen is the interval of time between infection by a pathogen and detection of that pathogen by a specific testing method. Nucleic acid testing (NAT) shortens the window period for HIV, HCV and HBV relative to serology and therefore may decrease the risk of transmitting disease from a serologically negative donor(Humar, Morris et al. 2010). For example, NAT for HBV can detect infections 21.8-36 days earlier when compared to standard serologic assays(Singer, Kucirka et al. 2008). Although routine NAT of potential organ donors may seem logical, it has not been rigorously studied. NAT is costly and may be logistically challenging. Most importantly, false-positive results may lead to unnecessary loss of uninfected organs(Humar, Morris et al. 2010). A 2008 survey of the 58 U.S. organ procurement organizations (OPOs) documented that 47% performed NAT on all potential donors(Orlowski, Alexander et al. 2009). Another 28% performed NAT on a subset of donors, usually based on the identification of behaviors thought to increase the risk of infection. OPOs tested for different pathogens using different assays, platforms and confirmatory algorithms with varied turn-around times and testing volumes. Some OPOs also noted geographic challenges in NAT accessibility, thus contributing to the varied practices observed. The turnaround time for NAT is also highly variable, ranging from 12-36 hours. Time is critical in organ donation, since delays in organ recovery and prolongation of cold-ischemic time affects organ utilization and posttransplant function. Current guidelines state that there is insufficient evidence to recommend routine NAT for HIV, HCV and HBV as the standard of care for screening all potential organ donors (level III evidence), but should be considered to reduce the risk of disease transmission and potentially increase organ utilization in increased-risk donors (level II evidence)(Humar, Morris et al. 2010).

Organs from donors with specified known viral hepatitis can be considered for specific recipients. For example, donors infected with HBV who are positive for IgG antibodies against hepatitis B core antigen (anti-HBc) can be used for some recipients who have been vaccinated or who were previously infected with HBV, provided there is prophylaxis with anti-HBV antiviral agents(Fabrega, Garcia-Suarez et al. 2003; Seehofer and Berg 2005; Prakoso, Strasser et al. 2006). The use of organs infected with HCV can generally be used in other HCV-infected recipients, although this practice remains somewhat controversial(Peek and Reddy 2007).

2.1.2 Recipient-derived infections and screening recommendations

Active viral hepatitis in solid organ transplant recipients is common and efforts should be made to detect and eradicate the infection prior to transplantation, since immunosuppression will exacerbate the infectious process. Prior to the era of antiviral prophylaxis (late 1980s), 80% of patients experienced HBV reinfection after liver transplantation(O'Grady, Smith et al. 1992). However, with the advent of hepatitis B immunoglobulin (HBIG) and the first oral antiviral agent for HBV, lamivudine, in the mid-late 1990s, graft reinfection has become the exception rather than the rule (Buti, Mas et al. 2007; Coffin and Terrault 2007). In contrast, the course of HCV infection after liver transplantation remains discouraging. Since effective antiviral therapies are lacking, recipients are uniformly reinfected by HCV, with outcomes determined by the viral strain, the presence or absence of previous immunity, and the response to antiviral therapy(Lake 2006; Gurusamy, Tsochatzis et al. 2010).

Similar to donor screening, recipient screening is based on the epidemiologic history and serologic testing of the recipient. At our institution, all potential solid organ transplant recipients are screened with serologic testing for antibodies to CMV, EBV, HSV, VZV, HBV (HBsAg, anti-HBs), and HCV. In addition, special serologic testing using nucleic acid assays based on epidemiologic risk factors and recent exposures is performed (e.g. HBV or HCV viral load).

2.1.3 Nosocomial-derived infections

Although rare, patients waiting for organ transplantation may become infected with hepatitis viruses via blood transfusion or hemodialysis. A 2010 study on HBV in donated blood suggests that the risk is about 1 in every 350,000 units or less (Zou, Dorsey et al. 2010). The transmission of HCV via transfusion currently stands at about a rate of 1 in 2 million units(Dwyre, Holland et al. 2008).

In the hemodialysis setting, cross-contamination to patients via environmental surfaces, supplies, equipment, multiple-dose medication vials and staff members is mainly responsible for both HBV and HCV transmission. The incidence and prevalence of HBV in hemodialysis centers have dropped markedly as a result of isolation strategies for HBsAg positive patients, the implementation of infection control measures and the introduction of HBV vaccine(Edey, Barraclough et al. 2010). The incidence and prevalence of HCV infection among hemodialysis patients remain higher than the corresponding general population.

2.2 Role of immunosuppression

Several immunosuppressant protocols are associated with an increased risk of viral activation. For example, induction therapy with T-lymphocyte-depleting antibodies such as the CD25-receptor antibodies (Interleukin-2 (IL-2) receptor antagonists, basiliximab or daclizumab) are associated with increased reactivation of HHV-6 (Acott, Crocker et al. 2004). In addition, alemtuzumab (Campath-1H, anti-CD52 monoclonal antibody) induction has been associated with rapidly progressive HCV recurrence in addition to an increased risk of viral infections posttransplant compared to controls (Marcos, Eghtesad et al. 2004; Levitsky, Thudi et al. 2011). On the other hand, the IL-2 receptor antagonists have been shown to result in lower rates of CMV infection, especially in kidney transplant recipients (Webster, Ruster et al. 2010). Finally, OKT3, a murine-depleting monoclonal anti-CD3 antibody is currently used in the setting of steroid-resistant rejection and has been associated with a higher risk of development post-transplant lymphoproliferative disorder (PTLD) which is commonly an EBV-related lymphoma(Opelz and Dohler 2004).

3. Common causes of viral hepatitis in solid organ transplant recipients

The issues related to viral hepatitis in organ transplant recipients are complex, and the approach to management is highly dependent on the organ transplanted. The approach to liver transplant patients is significantly different from that of nonhepatic organ transplant recipients of viral hepatitis and thus the discussion will be presented based on the type of organ (liver versus non-liver) transplanted.

3.1 Hepatitis B

HBV is a DNA virus that is transmitted parenterally, sexually, and perinatally, and leads to chronic infection in 1.25 million persons in the United States and 350 to 400 million persons worldwide. HBV infection accounts annually for 4000 to 5500 deaths in the United States and 1 million deaths worldwide from cirrhosis, liver failure, and hepatocellular carcinoma (HCC)(Dienstag 2008).

Chronic HBV infection can be divided into several phases(Lok 2002). Initially, there is an immune tolerance phase, in which HBV replicates actively but host immune responses to the virus are minimal. After 20–30 years, the immune tolerance phase evolves to an immune clearance phase in which HBV-specific cellular immunity becomes active, leading to inflammation and damage of hepatocytes. Levels of HBV viremia decrease drastically after this phase, and HBV infection then becomes residual. Nevertheless, the infection may reactivate in some patients(Lok 2002). HBV replication correlates with the presence of hepatitis B e antigen (HBeAg). Prolonged HBeAg sero-positivity or high HBV viral load is associated with prolonged liver injuries and a higher risk of HCC(Yang, Lu et al. 2002). The immune responses during HBV infection are responsible to the injuries in the liver (Bertoletti and Gehring 2007).

3.1.1 HBV in the Liver Transplant recipient

3.1.1.1 Epidemiology & specific risk factors

Fulminant hepatitis and cirrhosis caused by HBV are important indications for LT accounting for ~10% of all LT in the United States. Vaccination against HBV has dramatically reduced the prevalence of HBV infection in candidates for LT, but it remains elevated in patients from developing countries(Chen 2009).

Prior to the era of antiviral prophylaxis, 80% of patients experienced HBV reinfection after LT, resulting in a 50% two-year posttransplant mortality(Todo, Demetris et al. 1991). Although the major source of viral replication (the liver) is removed, circulating virions in extrahepatic sites, such as peripheral blood mononuclear cells, can reinfect the newly transplanted liver soon after liver transplant(Feray, Zignego et al. 1990). In the mid 1990s, Lamivudine (LAM), the first oral antiviral agent for HBV, in addition to hepatitis B immunoglobulin (HBIG) revolutionized the treatment of HBV. Long-term high-dose HBIG combined with LAM can reduce HBV recurrence to less than 10%(Chen, Yi et al. 2010).

However, combined treatment with HBIG and LAM is sometimes unable to control recurrent HBV infection. Recurrent graft infection may lead to rapid disease progression and even death within the first year after LT(Kennedy and Alexopoulos 2010). While uncommon, viral resistance to antiviral therapy and HBIG may cause HBV-related graft dysfunction(Cooreman, Leroux-Roels et al. 2001). Additional risk factors for recurrence include high viral load (> 2×10^4 IU/mL [10^5 copies/mL]) at the time of LT, high levels of immunosuppression, HBeAg positivity and prophylaxis noncompliance. Recurrence is less common in patients undergoing LT for fulminant HBV or those with concurrent hepatitis delta virus (HDV) infection as such patients typically have lower viral loads(Marzano, Gaia et al. 2005). The aggressive clinical course is probably due to stimulation of viral replication and direct cytotoxicity of HBV under immunosuppressive therapy(Jiang and Yan 2010). Therefore, suppression of HBV replication is paramount to prevent disease progression in the transplanted liver.

3.1.1.2 Diagnosis

HBV recurrence is typically defined as the reappearance of HBsAg after LT. This is generally associated with detectable HBV DNA in the blood, although viremia may also occur in the absence of HBs-antigenemia. HBV DNA has been detected in the serum, liver and peripheral blood mononuclear cells of HBsAg-negative patients on long-term prophylaxis using sensitive polymerase chain reaction (PCR)-based techniques(Roche, Feray et al. 2003). The clinical significance of these observations remain uncertain but is likely because of persistent occult HBV infection which may be sensitive to changes in HBV prophylaxis or modulation of immunosuppression.

Once activation of virus replication takes place, aggressive hepatitis and subsequent rapid development of liver failure may develop (a syndrome described as fibrosing cholestatic hepatitis, or FCH). FCH is defined as a rapidly progressive liver disease with cholestasis, jaundice, hepatic fibrosis, and liver failure, often complicated by sudden and severe multiorgan dysfunction(Angus, Locarnini et al. 1995). With appropriate post-LT prophylaxis, FCH is an extremely rare condition and should not be seen unless there is patient nonadherence. Retransplantation has been performed in patients with FCH, but those who have rapid liver failure shortly after OLT have poor survival (Kim, Wiesner et al. 1999).

Monitoring protocols for HBV recurrence after LT vary among transplant centers. HBsAg and DNA should be performed at least every 3 months even with HBIG and oral antiviral therapy. Although newer, more potent antiviral agents or combination therapy are associated with a lower potential for drug resistance, currently there are insufficient data to allow for less frequent monitoring(Levitsky and Doucette 2009). Persistent detection of HBV DNA levels of >3 log copies/mL during prophylaxis therapy indicates HBV recurrence and warrants a change in HBV therapy.

3.1.1.3 Treatment

Pretransplant: Antiviral therapy prior to LT, particularly if HBV DNA can be reduced to undetectable levels (or at least < 2 X 10^4 IU/mL), reduces the risk of HBV recurrence. Seven drugs are licensed in the United States for the treatment of HBV infection: interferon alfa (IFNα), pegylated interferon alfa-2a (Peg-IFNα), lamivudine (LAM), adefovir dipivoxil (ADV), entecavir (ETV), telbivudine, and tenofovir (TDF)(Dienstag 2008). The use of IFN, which requires injections daily or thrice weekly, has been supplanted by long-acting Peg-IFN, which is injected once weekly. A detailed discussion of pre-transplant HBV therapy is beyond the scope of this chapter. In general, therapy should be with a potent nucleos(t)ide analogues or combination therapy and based on published guidelines(Bhattacharya and Thio 2010; Alberti and Caporaso 2011). IFN therapy is not recommended in decompensated cirrhotic patients given the risk of precipitating hepatitis flares and further decompensation(Levitsky and Doucette 2009).

Posttransplant recurrence: HBV infection after LT is usually the result of failed prophylaxis (see *prophylaxis/prevention),* either due to noncompliance or the development of drug- or HBIG-resistant HBV infection. The management strategies are the same regardless of the reason for HBV infection, but the choice of antiviral agents will be dictated by whether the virus is wild-type or mutant.

In the pre-LAM era, IFN-α was a common therapeutic option for patients with recurrent HBV infection after LT. However, with the advent of LAM, it has not been used as a first-line treatment drug. Patients using IFN-α have a lower efficacy and a higher risk of precipitating allograft rejection than those using LAM(Terrault, Holland et al. 1996). LAM has been used in the treatment of recurrent HBV infection, with an excellent safety profile in both compensated and decompensated cirrhotic patients(Perrillo, Rakela et al. 1999). However, the major factor limiting the use of LAM in the treatment of graft HBV infection after LT is the development of mutations in the thyrosine-methionine-aspartate-aspartate (YMDD) motif of the HBV DNA polymerase gene, which confers resistance to LAM. In non-immunosuppressed patients, the LAM resistance rate is 15%-20%, however LAM resistance is detected in as many as 45% immunosuppressed patients within the first year of treatment (Lai, Dienstag et al. 2003). Thus, although LAM therapy results in a loss of viral replication markers in serum, an improved hepatic biochemical profile and improvement or stabilization in liver histology, LAM resistance and its possible accompanying clinical deterioration have limited its long-term use in the treatment of recurrent HBV infection after LT(McCaughan, Spencer et al. 1999).

Adefovir dipivoxil (ADV), a nucleotide analog that selectively inhibits viral polymerases and reverse transcriptase, is effective against HBeAg-negative and positive cases and has an excellent activity against wild-type as well as LAM-resistant HBV strains(Perrillo, Schiff et al. 2000; Hadziyannis, Tassopoulos et al. 2003). Additionally, ADV plus LAM can achieve favorable outcomes of HBsAg seroconversion and undetectable HBV DNA in patients with *de novo* graft HBV infection and LAM resistance(Toniutto, Fumo et al. 2004). Mildly elevated serum creatinine level may occur after treatment with ADV, especially in combination with calcineurin inhibitors, but only a small number of patients require dose adjustment, and even discontinuance(Jiang and Yan 2010). However, renal function should be regularly monitored, with dose adjustments based on renal function, as necessary.

Entecavir (ETV), a very potent anti-HBV selective guanosine analogue, approved by the United States FDA in 2005, can also be used in the treatment of chronic HBV infection.

Unfortunately, few reports are available on ETV in treatment of recurrent HBV infection. Most data concerning its efficacy and safety are obtained from patients without LT. ETV is superior to LAM or ADV in rendering HBV-DNA undetectable and has a very good resistance profile, with <2% cumulative 5-year resistance rate in nucleos(t)ide-naïve chronic HBV patients(Papatheodoridis, Manolakopoulos et al. 2008). In addition, it lacks the nephrotoxicity that can be seen with ADV, making it an attractive option. However, the high probability of resistance with long-term ETV documented in non-transplant patients with LAM resistance suggests this ETV is not a good option for LAM-resistant cases post-transplant(Tenney, Rose et al. 2007). In cases without LAM resistance, ETV could be used due to its great potency, high genetic barrier and absence of nephrotoxicity.
Tenofovir disoproxil fumarate (TDF), a nucleotide analogue has excellent antiviral activity against both wild-type and LAM-resistant HBV both *in vitro* and *in vivo*(Ying, De Clercq et al. 2000; Kuo, Dienstag et al. 2004; Lada, Benhamou et al. 2004; Marcellin, Heathcote et al. 2008). Furthermore, TDF shows a stronger antiviral effect than ADV on LAM-resistant HBV(van Bommel, Zollner et al. 2006). In addition, TDF plus LAM can safely and markedly suppress HBV replication in patients with resistance to or non-response to ADV(Choe, Kwon et al. 2008). Finally, in pretransplant chronic HBV patients with resistance to both LAM and ADV, TDF retains significant activity against HBV although this appears diminished in comparison with studies of naïve patients(Patterson, George et al. 2011). Only two studies are available on the application of TDF in the treatment of recurrent HBV infection after LT(Neff, Nery et al. 2004). An additional pilot study suggests that combination therapy with ETV-TDF may be more effective than monotherapy for HBV recurrence following LT(Jimenez-Perez, Saez-Gomez et al. 2010). Finally, TDF has significant renal tubular toxicity, and in more severe cases, patients can develop Fanconi syndrome (which is characterized by tubular proteinuria, amino aciduria, phosphaturia, glycosuria, and bicarbonate wasting [leading to metabolic acidosis] or acute kidney injury. Renal toxicity is especially prevalent after liver transplant in the setting of immunosuppressant medications that also effect renal function. Although TDF can significantly decrease LAM-resistant HBV variant replication after LT, further studies are needed to determine its efficacy and safety profile with a long follow-up time and a large cohort of patients.

3.1.1.4 Prevention/prophylaxis

Advances in antiviral prophylaxis have dramatically improved the outcome of transplantation in HBV-infected recipients. HBIG, a polyvalent immunoglobulin with a high titer of anti-HBs, binds to intracellular and circulating virions to prevent graft infection and quickly became the standard of care at most centers worldwide that provide LT. The high cost of HBIG ($30–50,000/yr), the inconvenience of ongoing IV infusions and the need for continued anti-HBs monitoring have stimulated discussions about alternative prophylaxis therapies(Gish and McCashland 2006). LAM monotherapy improves the rate of recurrence over no prophylaxis, although the development of resistance results in recurrence in 10-50% of patients within 1-3 years after LT(Perrillo, Rakela et al. 1999; Zheng, Chen et al. 2006). In contrast to monotherapy, combination therapy with IV HBIG and LAM is highly efficacious in preventing graft infection (<10%)(Markowitz, Martin et al. 1998; Dumortier, Chevallier et al. 2003; Gane, Angus et al. 2007). Samuel et al. was the first to describe the use of hepatitis B immunoglobulin (HBIG) in a large clinical trial to prevent recurrent liver disease after LT in patients with liver failure due to HBV infection(Samuel, Muller et al. 1993).

One major question to answer has been to discover if and when patients can be discontinued from HBIG therapy and maintained on antiviral therapy alone. Notably, the recurrence rate of HBV infection in the liver graft exceeds 60% with short-term HBIG monotherapy (< 6 months), but is < 10% if HBIG is stopped more than 6 months to 1 year after LT with continuation of a nucleoside such as LAM(Dodson, de Vera et al. 2000). In addition, the use of low-dose intramuscular HBIG is also evolving(Yao, Osorio et al. 1999; Yan, Yan et al. 2006; Gane, Angus et al. 2007). Although it has not yet been defined who can safely discontinue HBIG therapy, the best candidates are probably patients with undetectable HBV DNA before LT who use combination therapy with medications that have low risk of resistance.

In addition to HBIG + LAM prophylaxis, low recurrence rates have also been demonstrated in patients given combination oral antiviral therapy (LAM + ADV) prior to LT and who continued therapy post-LT with or without the use of postoperative HBIG therapy(Schiff, Lai et al. 2003). In addition, cost modeling has demonstrated that LAM + ADV may be much cheaper because of the high cost of HBIG(Dan, Wai et al. 2006). However, there are currently insufficient data to recommend post-LT prophylaxis with nucleos(t)ide analogues alone in the absence of HBIG. Similar to treatment of recurrent HBV, the choice of prophylaxis for HBV should be based on antiviral exposure history, resistance testing and the principles of HBV therapy pre-LT.

Finally, all HBV uninfected, nonimmune LT candidates should be vaccinated for HBV as early as possible pre-LT. The percentage of patients who successfully seroconvert, however is suboptimal (16-62%), even with double dose regimans, and many (37%-73%) lose antibodies to HBsAg within the first year following LT(Levitsky and Doucette 2009).

3.1.1.5 Anti-HBc positive donors

Donors who are anti-HBc positive pose a significant risk (ranging 34–86%) of transmitting HBV infection to liver transplant recipients without prophylaxis(Nery, Nery-Avila et al. 2003). Oral antiviral therapy is effective prophylaxis, with or without HBIG, in recipients of these organs and should be continued indefinitely post-transplant, unless HBV DVA negativity can be confirmed in the serum and liver tissue of the donor(Nery, Nery-Avila et al. 2003).

Rarely, despite prophlyaxis, late HBV infection with antiviral-resistant HBV has been described. The role of HBIG is not defined and should not have any specific benefit because the liver is already infected and there is no benefit to binding circulating virus(Gish and McCashland 2006). Because patients have developed fulminant HBV in this setting, even with the use of LAM, combination therapy or drugs with a high barrier to resistance may be the best option. The role of routine HBsAg and/or HBV DNA monitoring in recipients of anti-HBc-positive grafts is unclear; however unexplained aminotransferase elevation should be investigated with HBsAg and HBV DNA to rule out *de novo* HBV infection(Levitsky and Doucette 2009).

3.1.2 HBV in other solid organ transplants

3.1.2.1 Epidemiology & specific risk factors

With current infection control practices and the institution of widespread vaccination, the prevalence of chronic HBV in patients on hemodialysis has declined in developed countries and ranges between 0% and 7%(Burdick, Bragg-Gresham et al. 2003). In addition, acquisition of HBV on dialysis is now uncommon. In contrast, the epidemiology of HBV among dialysis patients in the less-developed world is not well known. There are scattered reports, typically single-center surveys, with rates of chronic HBsAg carriers ranging between 2% and 20%(Covic, Iancu et al. 1999; Vladutiu, Cosa et al. 2000; Carrilho, Moraes et al. 2004; Yakaryilmaz, Gurbuz et al. 2006). The higher HBV infection rates within dialysis units in the developing world can be attributed to several factors, such as the higher background prevalence of HBV in the general population, difficulties following infection control strategies against HBV such as "standard" precautions, vaccination against HBV, and blood screening. Many of these deficiencies are often attributable, at least in part, to a lack of financial and other resources(Fabrizi, Lunghi et al. 2002). Iatrogenic transmission of HBV has also been reported after transplantation of two stored vessel conduits from hepatitis-seropositive donors into seronegative kidney transplant recipients(MMWR 2011). The prevalence of chronic HBV in other nonhepatic transplant candidates has not been well studied, but likely mirrors the population prevalence(Wedemeyer, Pethig et al. 1998). Interestingly, in cardiac allograft recipients, HBV contamination can occur after transplantation and is related to nosocomial infection associated with the use of cardiac myotomes for myocardial biopsies. On the other hand, nosocomial transmission of HBV via blood transfusion is rare given the systematic screening of blood products for HBV, but, nevertheless, HBV is still the most frequent blood-borne infection (1/700,000)(Thompson, Perz et al. 2009).

Chronic HBV infection (HBsAg-positive) has been associated with an increased risk of death in renal transplant patients and is attributed to both progressive HBV-related disease as well as an increased risk of septic events(Correa, Rocha et al. 2003). Increased mortality, if it occurs, is usually seen ten years or more following renal transplantation. Contradictory results concerning the long-term outcomes of HBV infection in heart transplant recipients have been reported. Some authors have described a poor outcome, with cirrhosis occurring in more than 55% of patients within the first decade after transplantation, and 17% of patients dying of liver failure(Wedemeyer, Pethig et al. 1998). Others have reported little impact on short- or long-term survival (Lunel, Cadranel et al. 2000). However, more recent studies in renal and cardiac transplantation have demonstrated excellent outcomes in HBsAg-positive patients managed with nucleos(t)ide analogue therapy(Ko, Chou et al. 2001; Park, Yang et al. 2001; Potthoff, Tillmann et al. 2006; Ahn, Kim et al. 2007).

In nonhepatic solid organ transplant (SOT) recipients with markers of past HBV infection (HBsAg-negative; anti-HBc positive), there is a low risk (<5%) of HBV reactivation(Blanpain, Knoop et al. 1998). Although uncommon, when present, reactivation has been associated with rapid progression to cirrhosis and death(Knoll, Pietrzyk et al. 2005).

HBV uninfected, nonimmune, patients undergoing SOT may acquire donor derived HBV. The HBsAg-positive donor carries a high risk of transmission to recipients although satisfactory outcomes have been described with prophylaxis (see prevention/prophylaxis). The risk of HBV transmission from an anti-HBc-positive nonhepatic donor is significantly lower (<5%) than that of hepatic donors. Organs from anti-HBc-positive donors can be safely used with informed consent and appropriate strategies to prevent transmission (Levitsky and Doucette 2009).

3.1.2.2 Diagnosis

The diagnosis of HBV in nonhepatic SOT relies on the same serological and nucleic acid assays used in the nontransplant population(Lok 2002). Liver biopsy should be incorporated in the evaluation of renal transplant candidates with HBsAg because it is difficult, on clinical grounds alone, to estimate the severity of liver disease in uremic patients(Fabrizi, Lunghi et al. 2002). Administration of desmopressin acetate (DDAVP) at the time of biopsy should be considered to lessen the risk of bleeding caused by platelet dysfunction. A decision concerning transplant candidacy in HBsAg-positive patients should be based on both liver histology and evaluation of HBV replication by serum markers (i.e., HBeAg and HBV DNA). The absence of serum markers of replication before transplantation, however, does not preclude reactivation of HBV posttransplant and all patients should receive HBV prophylaxis (see Prophylaxis/Prevention).

3.1.2.3 Treatment

Nonhepatic SOT candidates with chronic HBV should be evaluated to determine the need for therapy prior to transplantation. If active replication is present (i.e., positive HBV DNA or HBeAg), antiviral therapy should be started to slow the progression of liver disease and should be based on published guidelines for the treatment of HBV(Bhattacharya and Thio 2010; Alberti and Caporaso 2011). If the initial histology shows more advanced fibrotic changes, a comprehensive evaluation should attempt to determine the likelihood of progression to decompensated cirrhosis. Although conventional wisdom has been that the presence of cirrhosis is an absolute contraindication to isolated nonhepatic SOT, an argument can be made that with effective antiviral therapy it is possible to abort progression of liver disease and presumably prevent hepatic decompensation post-transplant(Fabrizi, Lunghi et al. 2002).

Although antiviral therapy is not generally recommended for acute HBV in immunocompetent individuals given the extremely high (>85%) rate of spontaneous resolution, treatment of acute HBV may be appropriate in immunosuppressed individuals following transplant(Dulai, Higa et al. 1999). For reactivation of HBV, treatment with a potent nucleos(t)ide analogue, adjusted for renal function as needed, is preferred to limit the potential for future resistance. IFN-based therapy should be avoided as it is generally poorly tolerated in those with comorbid medical conditions and associated with a low rate of response in immunocomprised hosts.

As discussed previously, nucleos(t)ide analogues like ETV or TDF are recommended in the general population for the treatment of chronic HBV infection. They are more potent and have a higher genetic barrier than LAM or ADF. However, while the risk of resistance to ETV is low in treatment-naive patients, it may be as high as 51% at five years in LAM-resistant patients. TDF is more effective than ADF in the non-renal transplant population, is effective in LAM-resistant patients and does not lead to resistance after three years of treatment(Marcellin, Heathcote et al. 2008; Heathcote, Marcellin et al. 2011). TDF has a much lower renal toxicity than ADF and should be preferred in kidney transplant recipients.

3.1.2.4 Prevention/prophylaxis

As in liver transplantation, HBV uninfected, nonhepatic SOT candidates who are nonimmune should be vaccinated for HBV as early in the course of their disease as possible(Levitsky and Doucette 2009). However, vaccine immunogenicity is low in dialyzed patients (around 70%) and even lower in renal transplant recipients (30%) as compared to 90% in the general population(Keating and Noble 2003). Additionally, seroconversion rates decrease with declining renal function(DaRoza, Loewen et al. 2003). Factors related to a poor vaccine response can be acquired, such as ageing, or genetic, such as gender or the HLA

A1B8DR3 "non-responder" haplotype(Davila, Froeling et al. 2010). When the standard protocol is ineffective, the use of intensified protocols or intradermal injections can reinforce immunogenicity in hemodialyzed patients(Benhamou, Courouce et al. 1984; Nagafuchi, Kashiwagi et al. 1991). Finally, booster vaccinations can play an important role in improving immunogenicity, even in the absence of response to primary immunization: a booster injection in renal transplant recipients, vaccinated while on hemodialysis, has a global efficacy of 84%(Jungers, Devillier et al. 1994). There are limited data with regard to the efficacy of HBV vaccination in heart and lung transplant candidates; however small series suggest seroconversion rates of 45% and 53%, respectively(Hayney, Welter et al. 2003; Foster, Murphy et al. 2006).

The Kidney Disease: Improving Global Outcomes (KDIGO) guidelines recommend that all HBsAg-positive kidney transplant candidates and recipients receive prophylaxis with TDF, ETV or LAM to prevent reactivation; however, TDF and ETV are preferable to LAM to minimize the development of drug resistance(Kasiske, Zeier et al. 2010). Antiviral therapy should be continued indefinitely posttransplant.

In those with markers of past HBV infection (anti-HBc-positive), there is a low risk (<5%) of HBV reactivation(Knoll, Pietrzyk et al. 2005). Either antiviral prophylaxis or regular serologic monitoring should be employed to limit the risk associated with HBV reactivation(Levitsky and Doucette 2009). If nucleos(t)ide analogues are not used, recipients should undergo testing for HBsAg, HBV DNA and ALT every 1-3 months with antivirals initiated if HBsAg becomes positive or if HBV DNA progressively rises.

3.1.2.5 Anti-HBc positive donors

Recipients of an organ from a HBsAg positive donor, regardless of immune status, should receive combined prophylaxis with HBIG and a nucleos(t)ide analogue indefinitely(Chung, Feng et al. 2001). If the HBsAg and HBV DNA remain negative, consideration may be given to discontinuing HBIG 6-12 months posttransplant. In recipients of an organ from an anti-HBc positive donor, the risk of transmission is essentially eliminated if the recipient is immune and no further prophylaxis is needed(Chung, Feng et al. 2001; Levitsky and Doucette 2009). In HBV nonimmune recipients of an anti-HBc positive organ, prophylaxis with LAM (or other antiviral therapy) should be initiated. An assessment of HBV DNA in the donor may be used to further guide prophylaxis. If the donor HBV DNA is positive or unknown, prophylaxis should be continued with HBIG for at least 3-6 months or LAM for at least 12 months (Chung, Feng et al. 2001; Levitsky and Doucette 2009). If the donor is HBV DNA is negative, prophylaxis can be discontinued, but routine monitoring should continue with transaminases, HBsAg and HBV DNA every 3 to 6 months(Levitsky and Doucette 2009).

3.2 Hepatitis C

Hepatitis C Virus (HCV) affects more than 4 million people in the United States and more than 170 million people globally(Lauer and Walker 2001). The institution of blood-screening measures in developed countries has decreased the risk of transfusion-associated hepatitis to a negligible level, but new cases continue to occur mainly as a result of injection-drug use and, to a lesser degree, through other means of percutaneous or mucous-membrane exposure. Progression to chronic liver disease occurs in the majority of HCV-infected persons, and infection with the virus is a leading cause of liver transplantation worldwide.

HCV is an RNA virus that belongs to the flaviviridae family, hepciviridae genius; the most closely related flaviviruses viruses are hepatitis G virus, yellow fever virus, and dengue virus(Robertson, Myers et al. 1998). The natural targets of HCV are hepatocytes and, possibly, B lymphocytes(Zignego, De Carli et al. 1995; Okuda, Hino et al. 1999). Viral replication is extremely robust, and it is estimated that more than 10 trillion virion particles are produced per day, even in the chronic phase of infection(Neumann, Lam et al. 1998). Replication occurs through an RNA-dependent RNA polymerase that lacks a "proofreading" function, which results in the rapid evolution of diverse but related virions within an infected person and presents a major challenge with respect to immune-mediated control of HCV(Lauer and Walker 2001).

Six distinct but related HCV genotypes and multiple subtypes have been identified on the basis of molecular relatedness. In the United States and Western Europe genotypes 1a and 1b are most common, followed by genotypes 2 and 3. The other genotypes are virtually never found in these countries but are common in other areas, such as Egypt in the case of genotype 4, South Africa in the case of genotype 5, and Southeast Asia in the case of genotype 6. Knowledge of the genotype is important because it has predictive value in terms of the response to antiviral therapy, with better responses associated with genotypes 2 and 3 than with genotype 1 and 4(Poynard 2004).

3.2.1 HCV in the Liver Transplant recipient

3.2.1.1 Epidemiology & specific risk factors

End-stage liver disease due to HCV is the most common indication for LT in the United States and Europe(Adam, McMaster et al. 2003). HCV recurrence post-LT is essentially universal. The time course of HCV reinfection is faster than among immunocompetent individuals: histologically proven hepatitis C–related cirrhosis can be documented within a mean of 5 years after transplantation. For this reason, recipients with HCV-related liver disease show worse posttransplantation outcomes and greater mortality rates compared with HCV-negative recipients(Forman, Lewis et al. 2002). Fibrosing cholestatic hepatitis, similar to that seen in the early days of HBV transplantation, fortunately only occurs in a small percentage of patients. Once recurrent HCV cirrhosis occurs, 40% decompensate within 1 year, resulting in a 1- and 4-year patient survival of only 66% and 33%, respectively(Brown 2005). Retransplantation for HCV-induced graft failure is associated with particularly poor outcomes and might not be considered in higher risk recipients with advanced age, renal insufficiency, high MELD, deconditioned status and aggressive early (<1 year) HCV recurrence(Neff, O'Brien et al. 2004).

Risk factors for accelerated HCV recurrence are shown in Table 1. The strongest predictors of recurrence are immunosuppressive therapy for acute rejection, CMV infection, preservation injury and older recipient and donor age. Pulsed intravenous methylprednisolone treatment for acute cellular rejection is associated with transient 1–2 log increases in HCV RNA levels(Gane 2008). In addition to being proviral, treatment of acute cellular rejection with corticosteroids is associated with increased mortality and graft loss in LT recipients with HCV infection (relative risk = 2.7–2.9, $p = 0.04$)(Charlton, Ruppert et al. 2004). In general, induction therapy with either lymphocyte depleting or nondepleting (IL-2 inhibitors) antibodies does not appear to increase the risk of recurrence. However, the use of lymphocyte depleting antibodies for treatment of steroid-refractory rejection profoundly increases the risk of an aggressive HCV recurrence and FCH. HIV coinfection has recently emerged as an important predictor of poor survival among liver transplant recipients with HCV infection. One-year patient mortality attributable to HCV in coinfected recipients ranges between 27% and 54%. Factors associated with increased risk of post-LT mortality among HCV–HIV coinfected recipients include African-American recipient ethnicity, pre-LT MELD score of >20, intolerance of HAART therapy and higher pre-LT HCV level of viremia(de Vera, Dvorchik et al. 2006). Reduced response rates to treatment of HCV with IFN and ribavirin further attenuate post-LT outcomes in HIV–HCV coinfected liver transplant recipients.

Definite	Controversial	Not clearly associated
Acute rejection therapy intravenous steroids Lymphodepleting antibody	Corticosteroid therapy Use vs. complete avoidance Rapid vs. slow tapering	Induction therapy IL-2 antibody Lymphodepleting antibody
Donor Age	Viral load (> 1 X 10^6 copies/ml) at transplant	HCV+ donor
Recipient Age	Genotype (1b)	Live donor
Cytomegalovirus infection	Donation after cardiac death	Maintenance immunosuppression
Ischemia/reperfusion injury	HLA mismatch	
Diabetes Mellitus		
HIV coinfection		

Table 1. Risk factors for accelerated HCV recurrence after liver transplantation
Adapted from Levitsky & Doucette, Am J Transplantation 2009

More controversial and less clearly defined risks for recurrence include pre-LT viral load, HCV genotype (1b), donor/recipient HLA differences and the use of donors after cardiac death. The effects of different maintenance immunosuppressive agents and steroid tapering regimens are also quite controversisal. Although steroid sparing regimens appear to be safe, a large (n = 312) randomized controlled study, that included a steroid free arm of immunosuppression, has, to date, found no difference in the rate of recurrence of HCV nor in patient or graft survival between steroid free and steroid utilizing arms (Klintmalm, Washburn et al. 2007). Currently, there is no compelling basis for avoiding corticosteroids in the early postoperative period. Recent data also support a slow tapering schedule of steroids in HCV+ recipients to avoid precipitating a more aggressive early recurrence seen with rapid steroid withdrawal(Berenguer, Aguilera et al. 2006). The effect of calcineurin inhibitors on HCV recurrence post-LT has also been a topic of debate. In a prospective randomized controlled study of 495 recipients with HCV infection, no difference was seen in the histological recurrence rate of hepatitis C at 12 months post-LT between patients receiving cyclosporine versus tacrolimus (Levy, Grazi et al. 2006). However, a meta-analysis of studies comparing the two calcineurin inhibitors found a patient and graft survival benefit associated with tacrolimus as maintenance immunosuppression (graft loss: hazards ratio (HR) = 0.73, 95% CI = 0.61–0.86) (McAlister, Haddad et al. 2006). Interestingly, cyclosporine has well-recognized *in vitro* anti-HCV effects and may also have antiviral *in vivo* effects (Martin, Busuttil et al. 2004). In one small uncontrolled study of 8 liver transplant recipients with recurrence of HCV, conversion from tacrolimus to cyclosporine while receiving treatment with Peg-IFNα and ribavirin resulted in 5 patients becoming HCV RNA negative (Sugawara, Kaneko et al. 2006). This finding needs to be confirmed in a controlled fashion and currently data do not support a significant difference in recurrence rates with the use of cyclosporine versus tacrolimus. Other adjunctive agents, such as mycophenolate mofetil, rapamycin and azathioprine, have not been shown to definitively impact the risk of recurrence (Zekry, Gleeson et al. 2004; Bahra, Neumann et al. 2005; Wiesner, Shorr et al. 2005).

Finally, the effect of living donor liver transplant (LDLT) and HCV+ donors on recurrence has recently been elucidated. While early reports suggested a higher rate of recurrence following LDLT, subsequent data have dispelled these concerns(Garcia-Retortillo, Forns et al. 2004; Terrault, Shiffman et al. 2007). The use of HCV+ donors (without fibrosis) for HCV+ recipients also does not appear to impact recurrence rates (Arenas, Vargas et al. 2003; Peek and Reddy 2007). The use of genotype 1 HCV+ donors into nongenotype 1 recipients is, however, not recommended.

3.2.1.2 Diagnosis

HCV infection of the allograft occurs at the time of transplantation, with negative-strand HCV RNA detectable in the first postoperative week. There are three phases in the physiology of a transplant (resection or 'pre-anhepatic' phase, anhepatic phase and post-reperfusion phase). HCV RNA is cleared rapidly from serum during the anhepatic phase. Following reperfusion, the rate of decrease in HCV RNA accelerates, almost certainly reflecting HCV binding to its obligatory hepatic receptors(Watt, Veldt et al. 2009). HCV RNA levels typically increase rapidly from week 2 post-LT, peaking by the fourth postoperative month. At the end of the first postoperative year, HCV RNA levels are, on an average, 10–20-fold greater than pre-LT levels. Histological features of hepatitis develop in approximately 75% of recipients in the first 6 months following LT(Neumann, Berg et al. 2004). By the fifth postoperative year up to 30% have progressed to cirrhosis(Neumann, Berg et al. 2004). A small proportion of patients (4–7%), develop an accelerated course of liver injury (cholestatic hepatitis C, associated with very high levels of viremia) with subsequent rapid allograft failure. Early post-LT histology, for example at 1 year, has been consistently predictive of subsequent fibrosis progression.

Liver function test abnormalities are common in HCV+ recipients and do not reliably differentiate HCV recurrence from other etiologies (i.e. rejection). The "gold standard" for diagnosis of HCV recurrence is liver biopsy, which still may not be accurate in differentiating other causes of early graft dysfunction from HCV recurrence and may also inaccurately stage the degree of fibrosis (Skripenova, Trainer et al. 2007). While supportive evidence is not available, most centers perform protocol liver biopsies every 1-2 years post-LT to monitor for evidence of histological recurrence. Therapy is usually reserved for patients who develop biopsy-proven recurrence (grade 3 or stage 1-2 by METAVIR) (Wiesner, Sorrell et al. 2003).

The hepatic venous pressure gradient (HVPG), noninvasive blood tests or imaging are additional available supportive tests for evaluation of the development of fibrosis, which is a marker of disease severity, following liver transplant. While a direct correlation between HVPG measurements and fibrosis may not be present in LT recipients, an elevated HVPG by itself has been shown to predict progression to more advance disease and the development of portal hypertension, and declines with successful anti-HCV therapy(Blasco, Forns et al. 2006; Forns and Costa 2006). Liver stiffness measurement with transient elastography offers a higher sensitivity and positive predictive value for advanced fibrosis in HCV+ recipients in comparison to other clinical markers(Carrion, Navasa et al. 2006; Benlloch, Heredia et al. 2009). In addition, serum markers of fibrosis, such as hyaluronic acid, have been shown to have reasonable predictive value(Carrion, Fernandez-Varo et al. 2010). Overall, none of these tests appear to individually provide an accurate assessment of disease progression, supporting the need for further investigation into combined modalities or surrogate markers.

3.2.1.3 Treatment

Pretransplant: Patients with higher pre-LT HCV RNA titers experience greater mortality and graft loss rates than recipients with lower pre-LT HCV RNA titers(Charlton 2007). Pre-LT therapy in patients with advanced liver disease is limited by reduced patient tolerability and efficacy(Crippin, McCashland et al. 2002). While IFN based therapy is generally safe in compensated cirrhotic patients, it is poorly tolerated and often risky in decompensated patients with advanced liver disease (MELD>20, Child Turcotte Pugh (CTP) class C). Given the high frequency of serious adverse events (33%), among patients with more severe liver disease (CTP class B or C), the International Liver Transplant Society (ILTS) consensus panel concluded that treatment should be limited to cirrhotic patients with CTP score ≤ 7 or MELD score < 18, and is contraindicated when the CTP score is >11 or MELD score is >25.

In 2010, the phase III results of the first generation HCV nonstructural protein 3/4A protease inhibitors (PIs: boceprevir, telaprevir) were presented(Jacobson, McHutchison et al. 2010; Poordad, McCone et al. 2011). After a decade in which Peg-IFNα–ribavirin therapy was the only available option, triple therapy with HCV PIs in combination with Peg-IFNα–ribavirin is becoming the new standard of care. However, since IFN is still used, this therapy also cannot be given in decompensated cirrhosis.

Posttransplant: Two approaches to post-LT HCV recurrence have been identified: early, pre-emptive, treatment, to be started within weeks after liver transplantation (see *prevention/prophylaxis* below); and treatment of established recurrent HCV infection. The treatment of histologically proven HCV reinfection with pegylated (PEG)-IFN and ribavirin is, at present, the standard of care at most LT centers.

Treatment of histological recurrence is only successful in 20-30% of recipients and is associated with high rates (30-50%) of discontinuation due to intolerability(Beckebaum, Cicinnati et al. 2004; Kornberg, Kupper et al. 2007). A major limiting factor in achieving an acceptable SVR rate is the inability to reach target ribavirin doses due to the high prevalence of renal insufficiency in HCV+ LT recipients(Chalasani, Manzarbeitia et al. 2005). Although earlier studies reported high rates (21-35%) of IFN-induced allograft rejection, a recent randomized study of early post-LT prophylaxis and therapy did not demonstrate an increase in the risk of acute rejection(Chalasani, Manzarbeitia et al. 2005). Finally, although triple therapy (addition of a PI to Peg-IFNα–ribavirin) is becoming the new standard of care for pretransplant HCV, this treatment regimen is not approved in solid organ transplant recipients and has significant potential for drug interaction with immunosuppressive therapy. Recently, genetic variation in the region of the IL28B gene on chromosome 19, coding for IFN-λ3, has been demonstrated to be strongly associated with SVR in patients with genotype 1 chronic HCV infection who are treated with pegIFN plus RBV in the nontransplant setting(Ge, Fellay et al. 2009). Charlton et al. recently also confirmed this finding in a transplant population(Charlton, Thompson et al. 2011). Donor and recipient IL28B genotype were independently associated with SVR and IL28B recipient genotype was predictive of fibrosis stage, with TT genotype being associated with more rapid fibrosis.

3.2.1.4 Prevention/prophylaxis

On a theoretical basis, an early antiviral approach should warrant better results. However, it is currently not recommended for at least 3 reasons: (1) in the immediate postoperative period, the exposure of human leukocyte antigen (HLA) of the major histocompatibility complex (MHC) is maximized, thus increasing the risk of acute rejection episodes in cases of use of immunomodulatory agents; (2) the recipient is usually still recovering from a major surgical procedure; and (3) this policy would cause unnecessary therapy for a significant number of recipients (maybe up to 50%) who will never develop overt liver disease(Castedal, Felldin et al. 2005). PHOENIX was a large, randomized study designed to compare the efficacy, tolerability, and safety of prophylactic initiation (before significant histological recurrence) of Peg-IFN2α plus ribavirin within 26 weeks after LT versus initiation only upon HCV recurrence. SVR was achieved in 22% of treated patients, however on an intent-to-treat basis, significant HCV recurrence at 120 weeks was similar in the prophylaxis (61.8%) and observation arms (65.0%, $P = 0.725$). The most common adverse event was anemia leading to dose reduction in 70% of the patients. The authors concluded that because of the safety profile of Peg-IFN2α/ribavirin and the lack of a clear benefit in terms of HCV recurrence and patient or graft survival, routine use of prophylactic antiviral therapy is not warranted(Bzowej, Nelson et al. 2011). Similar findings have been demonstrated in smaller, randomized controlled trials(Chalasani, Manzarbeitia et al. 2005). Finally, Hepatitis C immunoglobulin (Civacir®, Nabi Biopharmaceuticals, Rockville, MD) has been shown to lower HCV RNA but does not eliminate HCV viremia or the risk of recurrence(Davis, Nelson et al. 2005). There is currently no vaccine available for primary HCV prevention.

3.2.2 HCV in other solid organ transplants

3.2.2.1 Epidemiology & specific risk factors

The prevalence of HCV infection in candidates for nonhepatic SOT varies by organ group. HCV infection is more frequent in renal transplant recipients and dialysis patients than in the general population and has a significant impact on the survival of these patients(Aroldi, Lampertico et al. 2005). The annual incidence of HCV infection in hemodialysis ranges from 0% to 2.4% with a prevalence ranging between 10% and 65% according to the geographical zone(Elamin and Abu-Aisha 2011). HCV transmission is predominantly related to failure to comply with universal hygiene rules; compliance with universal hygiene rules has eliminated nosocomial transmission of HCV, and transmission by dialysis equipment *per se* is today anecdotal(Fissell, Bragg-Gresham et al. 2004; Jadoul, Poignet et al. 2004). Isolation of HCV-infected patients or the use of dedicated dialysis machines are not recommended(KDIGO 2008). In heart transplant patients, the prevalence of HCV - mainly transmitted by transfusion or heart donation - is about 11-16% and appears to approximate the population prevalence (Lunel, Cadranel et al. 2000).

The impact of HCV on transplant outcomes has been studied most extensively in renal transplant recipients. In this group, the rate of HCV-related fibrosis progression has been shown to be accelerated when compared to immunocompetent individuals (Zylberberg, Nalpas et al. 2002). HCV infection decreases both patient and graft survival post renal transplant, with the greatest impact occurring 5 or more years following transplant (Mathurin, Mouquet et al. 1999). The 10-year survival is approximately 15% lower in HCV+

compared to HCV- renal transplant recipients. Overall, however, survival is improved compared to those patients who remain on dialysis and poor outcomes primarily occur in those with advanced fibrosis/cirrhosis at transplant. Renal transplant candidates and recipients with mild to moderate (METAVIR stage F2 or less) liver disease at baseline have a low risk of progression of liver disease(Kamar, Boulestin et al. 2005). HCV+ recipients of a renal allograft also have an increased risk of posttransplant diabetes, graft dysfunction and proteinuria(Meyers, Seeff et al. 2003).

There are no long-term studies regarding the impact of HCV on outcomes of thoracic organ, small bowel or pancreas recipients. However, current studies in these populations suggest that patient and graft survival is not affected by HCV status(Lunel, Cadranel et al. 2000; Cano, Almenar et al. 2007; Sahi, Zein et al. 2007). Based on the renal transplant literature, there is likely an increased risk of HCV-related death beyond 5 years posttransplant in other nonhepatic SOT; however, further studies are needed to clarify the risk. On the other hand, posttransplant renal disease is common among HCV-positive recipients of any organ.

3.2.2.2 Diagnosis

The diagnosis of HCV infection relies on the same serologic and nucleic acid testing investigations used in the nontransplant population. Initial screening for antibody to HCV should be done at the time of initial transplant assessment using a third-generation enzyme immunoassay (EIA). However, in transplant candidates or recipients with negative HCV serology and persistent unexplained liver enzyme abnormalities, qualitative HCV RNA testing to rule out false negative testing should be considered. In those with positive HCV serology, qualitative HCV RNA and genotype tests should be used to confirm current infection (see *Treatment*). Abdominal ultrasound is used for identification of complications of HCV-related disease such as ascites, portal hypertension and hepatocellular carcinoma (HCC).

In chronic HCV infection, the liver biopsy remains the "gold standard" for assessing the degree of hepatic inflammation and fibrosis as well as the prognosis of the disease. Specifically, transjugular liver biopsy with hepatic venous pressure gradient (HVPG) measurement is recommended over percutaneous liver biopsy. Recent studies suggest that the proportion of the liver biopsy specimen occupied by collagen (a marker of liver fibrosis) is correlated with the HVPG in liver transplant recipients with HCV infection, with or without cirrhosis, and represents a predictor of clinical decompensation(Blasco, Forns et al. 2006). Biopsy is recommended in the assessment of nonhepatic SOT candidates with chronic HCV to guide antiviral treatment decisions, identify those who may be considered for combined (with liver) transplant and those who are ineligible for nonhepatic SOT due to advanced liver disease(Doucette, Weinkauf et al. 2007).

3.2.2.3 Treatment

Pretransplant: Eradication of HCV before transplantation has several theoretical benefits. HCV is associated with worse patient and graft survival as well as an increased risk for post-transplant diabetes mellitus and de novo glomerulopathy. Eradication of HCV before transplant might mitigate some of these adverse outcomes(Cruzado, Casanovas-Taltavull et al. 2003; Casanovas-Taltavull, Baliellas et al. 2007). Furthermore, IFN therapy after transplantation is associated with reduced treatment response rates, a greater incidence of organ rejection, and impairment of renal function(Rostaing, Izopet et al. 1995). Thus, it is best if treatment can be undertaken before embarking on the solid organ transplant.

Results of treatment of HCV in patients who are on dialysis varies, with reasonable SVR rates ranging from 16% to 68% with PEG or standard IFN(Fabrizi, Bunnapradist et al. 2005). Patients with bridging fibrosis or compensated cirrhosis should undergo IFN-based therapy and may be listed for transplant if an SVR is achieved. Those with decompensated cirrhosis are generally not considered candidates for isolated renal transplant but may be considered for simultaneous liver-kidney (SLK) transplant. For HCV-infected patients on maintenance hemodialysis, the KDIGO guidelines suggest monotherapy with standard interferon that is dose-adjusted for a GFR of <15 ml/min per 1.73 m^2(KDIGO2008). Importantly, ribavirin remains contraindicated in patients with a GFR < 50 mL/min, despite small studies that have suggested that with close monitoring and dose reduction it may be safe for use(Mousa, Abdalla et al. 2004; van Leusen, Adang et al. 2008).

In heart transplant candidates, HCV therapy is contraindicated due to the adverse effect profile (i.e. worsening anemia, risk of heart failure, myocardial infarction, arrhythmia). Although there are no published data on the outcome of lung transplant in HCV-positive recipients, one small series has shown that selected lung transplant candidates can safely and effectively be treated for HCV prior to transplant(Doucette, Weinkauf et al. 2007).

Posttransplant: Generally, posttransplantation IFN therapy is contraindicated in recipients of SOT, other than liver allografts due to a high risk of precipitation of organ rejection from IFN therapy(Shu, Lan et al. 2004; Kamar, Ribes et al. 2006). There is well-documented evidence to support the theory that the liver allograft provides some level of immunologic protection to the kidney allograft(Calne, Davis et al. 1971; Rasmussen, Davies et al. 1995). As such, recent reports have demonstrated successful HCV treatment with Peg-IFN and ribavirin in SLK recipients without development of renal rejection on therapy, although data are limited to small numbers of patients(Montalbano, Pasulo et al. 2007; Mukherjee and Ariyarantha 2007; Van Wagner, Baker et al. 2009).

Due to the risk of precipitating rejection, IFN-based therapy should therefore be avoided in life-sustaining (e.g. heart, lung) transplants. However, successful therapy has been reported postrenal transplant and may be considered on a case-by-case basis in those with severe disease following careful review of the potential risks and benefits.

3.2.2.4 Prevention/prophylaxis

The prevalence of HCV infection has decreased significantly since the introduction of various preventive measures: systematic screening of blood and organ donations, use of erythropoietin and compliance with universal hygiene rules. No HCV vaccine is available at the present time.

As discussed previously, serologic screening of all SOT candidates should be performed prior to transplant. In those candidates who are positive for HCV, a liver biopsy should be performed to assess underlying disease activity and the stage of HCV-related liver disease, which is not predicted well by biochemical tests. This information can help to guide expected response rates as well as the aggressiveness of therapy. IFN therapy is associated with reasonable response rates in patients who are on dialysis, with frequent maintenance of response after renal transplantation. Given the lower patient and graft survival rates after renal transplantation in patients who are HCV positive compared with patients who are HCV negative, IFN should be considered for candidates for renal transplantation who have HCV and active viral replication. Those with decompensated cirrhosis should be considered for SLK transplant.

There is little available data regarding the management of heart and lung transplant candidates with chronic HCV, therefore the principles and data from the renal transplant population should be used to guide management. As mentioned previously, HCV therapy is contraindicated in heart transplant candidates due to the adverse side effect profile. Those with mild-to-moderate disease (METAVIR stage F0-F2) may be listed for transplant, while those with advanced HCV-related fibrosis or cirrhosis are generally not considered ideal candidates for cardiac transplantation(Steinman, Becker et al. 2001). In lung transplant, HCV positivity is generally considered a contraindication to transplant, however one small series has shown that selected lung transplant candidates can safely and effectively be treated for HCV prior to transplantation(Orens, Estenne et al. 2006).

3.3 Hepatitis D

Hepatitis delta virus (HDV) is a small, defective RNA virus that can only replicate in an individual who has coexistent HBV, either after simultaneous transmission of the two viruses (co-infection), or via superinfection of an established HBV carrier(Pascarella and Negro 2011). The distribution pattern of this virus, investigated by seroprevalence studies of anti-HDV in HBsAg-positive patients, is worldwide but not uniform(Rizzetto, Ponzetto et al. 1991). For example, 90% of HBV carriers are infected with both viruses in the Pacific Islands, whereas the rates decline to 8% in Italy and 5% in Japan. Current estimates suggest that 15–20 million people are infected with HDV(Farci 2003).

Like HBV, HDV is transmitted via the parenteral route through exposure to infected blood or body fluids, and tests in chimpanzees have shown that only a very small inoculum is sufficient to transmit infection(Ponzetto, Hoyer et al. 1987). Thus, transmission rates remain high in intravenous drug users and those with high risk sexual activities. Perinatal transmission of HDV is uncommon. Because of screening of blood products, new infections in hemophiliacs, blood transfusion recipients, and patients receiving hemodialysis are no longer seen in developed countries.

The development of anti-HDV antibodies is universal in individuals with HDV; therefore, every patient who is HBsAg positive should be tested for anti-HDV IgG antibodies, which persist even after the patient has cleared HDV infection. Although active HDV infection was diagnosed historically by the presence of anti-HDV IgM antibodies, it is now confirmed by the detection of serum HDV RNA with a commercially available sensitive real-time PCR assay(Mederacke, Bremer et al. 2010).

A third minor pattern of infection, the so-called helper-independent latent infection, has been reported in the liver transplant setting and is discussed briefly below(Ottobrelli, Marzano et al. 1991). Patients who undergo LT with HDV infection are interesting from the perspective that they often have low or very low serum levels of HBV (low replication) and have an overall high survival rate (>80%) after LT as a result of the "antiviral" effect of HDV on HBV replication(Samuel, Zignego et al. 1995). Suppression of HBV replication by HDV has historically led to better posttransplantation survival in coinfected patients(Lerut, Donataccio et al. 1999). As discussed previously, HBV infection of the grafted liver is usually prevented by administration of hepatitis B immunoglobulins and thus, hepatocytes may thus be infected with HDV alone. HDAg can be detected in the liver by immunohistochemistry before HBV recurrence, as the helper virus is only necessary for particle formation and not for viral replication(Kuo, Chao et al. 1989). HDV viremia (as determined by molecular hybridization) is only observed several months later, when residual HBV evades neutralization, thus allowing for HDV rescue and cell-to-cell spread(Ottobrelli, Marzano et al. 1991). This third pattern of infection has been revisited with the advent of more sensitive, reverse transcription (RT)-PCR-based techniques for detecting HDV RNA(Pascarella and Negro 2011).

The goal of treatment pre and post-transplant is to eradicate HDV together with HBV. HDV is considered eradicated when both HDV RNA in the serum and HDAg in the liver become persistently undetectable. However, it is only with HBsAg clearance that complete and definitive resolution is attained. Standard treatment is usually with IFN-α and has been shown to improve long-term clinical outcome and survival(Farci, Roskams et al. 2004). However, Peg-IFNα is still insufficient to cure the majority of chronic hepatitis D patients. In a prospective trial, only 21% of patients achieved HDV RNA negativity(Niro, Ciancio et al. 2006). Alternative treatments have been tested, also with limited results. Antivirals such as lamivudine, adefovir dipivoxil, famciclovir and entecavir, have been shown to have some efficacy against HBV but no efficacy against HDV either in monotherapy or in combination with IFNα(Yurdaydin, Bozkaya et al. 2002; Niro, Ciancio et al. 2005; Hynicka, Yunker et al. 2010; Wedemeyer, Yurdaydin et al. 2011). Ribavirin has been shown to inhibit HDV replication *in vitro* but is ineffective *in vivo,* even if associated with Peg-IFNα(Rasshofer, Choi et al. 1991; Garripoli, Di Marco et al. 1994; Niro, Ciancio et al. 2006). Most transplant centers use a peri- and post-LT protocol that includes the use of HBIG and a nucleos(t)ide analogue to minimize the risk of HBV reactivation, although these two treatments will have no effect on HDV replication. There are currently no published reports of HDV recurrence following solid organ transplant.

3.4 Hepatitis E

3.4.1 Epidemiology & specific risk factors

Hepatitis E, caused by hepatitis E virus (HEV), was unknown as a disease entity until 1980 during an outbreak of acute viral hepatitis in the Kashmir Valley, India, with 275 clinical cases in small villages with a common water source(Khuroo 1980). In the initial years after its discovery, it was believed to be a common cause of sporadic and epidemic waterborne acute hepatitis in, and limited to, developing countries, primarily in Asia and Africa. However, in recent years, the host range, geographical distribution and modes of transmission of this virus, and clinical presentations of this infection have been shown to be much broader than were previously believed(Purcell and Emerson 2008; Aggarwal 2011).

The virus has four genotypes; of these, genotypes 1 and 2 are known to infect only humans, whereas genotypes 3 and 4 primarily infect other mammals, particularly pigs, but occasionally cause human disease(Lu, Li et al. 2006). The disease is characterized by a particularly severe course and high mortality among pregnant women(Navaneethan, Al Mohajer et al. 2008). In persons with pre-existing chronic liver disease, HEV superinfection can present as acute-on-chronic liver disease and can lead to liver decompensation and death. In non-endemic regions, chronic infection with genotype 3 HEV, which may progress to liver cirrhosis, has been reported among immunosuppressed hosts—including heart, kidney, kidney-pancreas and liver transplant recipients(Kamar, Mansuy et al. 2008; Haagsma, Niesters et al. 2009). There are no published reports of HEV in lung or small bowel transplant recipients.

Anti-HEV IgG antibodies are present in 16.6% of blood donors in France and in 6–16% of renal transplant recipients(Mansuy, Abravanel et al. 2009)(Kamar, Mansuy et al. 2008;

Mansuy, Abravanel et al. 2009). Approximately 60% of SOT patients infected with HEV will develop chronic hepatitis, and up to 15% will develop cirrhosis(Kamar, Garrouste et al. 2011). The use of tacrolimus rather than cyclosporine A and low platelet count have been reported as the main independent factors associated with chronic HEV infection after SOT(Kamar, Garrouste et al. 2011). Factors determining the severity of illness caused by HEV infection are not fully understood. These could include host factors or viral factors. Of these, host factors, in particular pregnancy, age and pre-existing liver disease clearly appear to be important(Aggarwal 2011). In addition, host immune response may also play a role. In a report from Japan, patients with genotype 4 HEV infection were found to have more severe illness than those who had infection with genotype 3 virus(Ohnishi, Kang et al. 2006). All patients with chronic HEV infection reported to date have been related to genotype 3 virus; no cases of chronic hepatitis E caused by infection with genotypes prevalent in high-endemic countries, namely genotype 1 and 2, have been described.

3.4.2 Diagnosis

The diagnosis of HEV infection in immunosuppressed individuals is not straightforward. Most patients have no symptoms, and clinically evident jaundice is rare. Immunosuppressed SOT recipients also have a lower degree of transaminase elevation (ALT 100 to 300 IU/L). The diagnosis of HEV infection is confirmed by serology and/or molecular techniques. However, diagnosis of HEV is limited by the lack of high sensitivity commercial assays for detecting HEV RNA and reliance on anti-HEV immunoglobulin M (IgM) antibody testing(Drobeniuc, Meng et al. 2010). Serologic testing for anti-HEV antibodies has a significant false-negative rate in immunosuppressed patients, so negative results should be treated with caution(Kamar, Garrouste et al. 2011). No serologic tests to diagnose HEV infection have been approved for commercial use in the United States though several tests are available for research purposes(CDC 2010).

3.4.3 Treatment

Data are currently lacking regarding the treatment of chronic HEV infection in SOT recipients. Peg-IFN seems to have some efficacy but must be used with caution because of the risk of graft rejection(Kamar, Rostaing et al. 2010). Reduction of immunosuppression may be helpful. In one study nearly one-third of patients who were chronically infected with HEV achieved viral clearance after dose reduction of immunosuppressive therapy, and this was mainly due to the reduction of T cell therapy(Kamar, Garrouste et al. 2011). Small studies have reported that ribavirin has promising efficacy in immunocompromised patients with chronic HEV infection, including kidney and heart recipients(Kamar, Rostaing et al. 2010; Mallet, Nicand et al. 2010; Chaillon, Sirinelli et al. 2011) .

3.4.4 Prevention/prophylaxis

Two recombinant vaccine candidates, the rHEV vaccine expressed in baculovirus and the HEV 239 vaccine, expressed in Escherichia coli, have been successfully evaluated in Phase II/III trials(Shrestha, Scott et al. 2007; Zhu, Zhang et al. 2010). The HEV 239 vaccine remains under development and is based on HEV genotype 1, the endemic form of HEV. However, no data are yet available on the safety and efficacy of HEV 239 in patients with chronic liver disease and in immunocompromised individuals. The vaccine has not been investigated for immunuity against zoonotic HEV genotype 3 infection, which currently represents the main

clinical challenge to immunocompromised patients in Europe and the USA(Wedemeyer and Pischke 2011).
The prevention of transmission of HEV is based on respect of hygiene rules, including the adequate cooking of meat. There is no systematic screening of HEV infection for blood donation. Although cases of blood-borne transmission of HEV have been described, the risk of parenteral transmission appears to be very low, as for hepatitis A virus(Franco, Giambi et al. 2003). Of note, following successful clearance of HEV, no reactivation has been observed following SOT(Legrand-Abravanel, Kamar et al. 2011).

4. Challenges and new advancements in the management of hepatotropic infections

Basic research, as well as the development of drugs and vaccines targeting human hepatotropic pathogens, has been handicapped by the lack of robust in vitro and in vivo platforms that mimic human liver biology and disease susceptibility. For example, despite prolonged viremia in mice models, none of the commonly observed sequelae associated with HBV or HCV infections in humans, namely fibrosis or HCC, have been observed in mouse models. However, the recent development of human liver-chimeric mice is evolving and appears promising(de Jong, Rice et al. 2010). Trials are ongoing to optimize the efficacy of available treatment options, for example, the use of protease inhibitors in combined therapy for HCV. In general, therapy for hepatotropic viruses is limited by the use of a few drugs that cause significant toxicities often resulting in dose adjustments and thus less efficacious regimens. Continuous efforts to improve treatment options available for viral hepatitis following solid organ transplant are urgently needed as viral hepatitis is a largely underestimated disease with an enormous impact on post-transplantation outcomes.
Finally, emerging concepts of individualized immunosuppression may result in a decreased incidence of overall infection following solid organ transplant.(Sarwal, Benjamin et al. 2011). The transplant community is putting significant effort into finding/solving the "Holy Grail" of transplantation: true, donor-specific tolerance (free of chemical immunosuppressive agents). One of the main questioned topics related to immunologic tolerance is whether the most realistic achievable ultimate goal is "true tolerance," with no maintenance immunosuppressive agents whatsoever or to achieve the status of "prope/almost tolerance," with minimal or non-toxic maintenance drug therapy (Scherer, Banas et al. 2007). In order to achieve either of these goals, an effective clinical-tolerance monitoring assay to identify and predict possibly tolerant transplant recipients who could possible be weaned off immunosuppressive agents is yet to be found.

5. Conclusions

Viral hepatitis has a significant impact on transplantation outcomes. HBV and HCV are the most common causes of viral hepatitis following SOT and HEV is emerging as a significant cause of chronic hepatitis in industrialized nations. The interaction of infection and immunosuppression is central to understanding of risk and pathogenesis of various hepatropic viruses. Future studies to address prevention and improved treatment modalities both pre- and post-SOT are needed.

6. References

(2008). "KDIGO clinical practice guidelines for the prevention, diagnosis, evaluation, and treatment of hepatitis C in chronic kidney disease." Kidney Int Suppl(109): S1-99.

(2011). "Potential transmission of viral hepatitis through use of stored blood vessels as conduits in organ transplantation--Pennsylvania, 2009." MMWR Morb Mortal Wkly Rep 60(6): 172-174.

Acott, P. D., J. F. S. Crocker, et al. (2004). "Simulect and HHV-6 in pediatric renal transplantation." Transplantation proceedings 36(2): S483-S486.

Adam, R., P. McMaster, et al. (2003). "Evolution of liver transplantation in Europe: report of the European Liver Transplant Registry." Liver Transpl 9(12): 1231-1243.

Aggarwal, R. (2011). "Clinical presentation of hepatitis E." Virus Res.

Aggarwal, R. (2011). "Hepatitis E: Historical, contemporary and future perspectives." J Gastroenterol Hepatol 26 Suppl 1: 72-82.

Ahn, H. J., M. S. Kim, et al. (2007). "Clinical outcome of renal transplantation in patients with positive pre-transplant hepatitis B surface antigen." J Med Virol 79(11): 1655-1663.

Alberti, A. and N. Caporaso (2011). "HBV therapy: guidelines and open issues." Dig Liver Dis 43 Suppl 1: S57-63.

Angus, P. W., S. A. Locarnini, et al. (1995). "Hepatitis B virus precore mutant infection is associated with severe recurrent disease after liver transplantation." Hepatology 21(1): 14-18.

Arenas, J. I., H. E. Vargas, et al. (2003). "The use of hepatitis C-infected grafts in liver transplantation." Liver Transpl 9(11): S48-51.

Aroldi, A., P. Lampertico, et al. (2005). "Natural history of hepatitis C virus infection in adult renal graft recipients." Transplant Proc 37(2): 940-941.

Bahra, M., U. I. Neumann, et al. (2005). "MMF and calcineurin taper in recurrent hepatitis C after liver transplantation: impact on histological course." Am J Transplant 5(2): 406-411.

Beckebaum, S., V. R. Cicinnati, et al. (2004). "Combination therapy with peginterferon alpha-2B and ribavirin in liver transplant recipients with recurrent HCV infection: preliminary results of an open prospective study." Transplant Proc 36(5): 1489-1491.

Benhamou, E., A. M. Courouce, et al. (1984). "Hepatitis B vaccine: randomized trial of immunogenicity in hemodialysis patients." Clin Nephrol 21(3): 143-147.

Benlloch, S., L. Heredia, et al. (2009). "Prospective validation of a noninvasive index for predicting liver fibrosis in hepatitis C virus-infected liver transplant recipients." Liver Transpl 15(12): 1798-1807.

Berenguer, M., V. Aguilera, et al. (2006). "Significant improvement in the outcome of HCV-infected transplant recipients by avoiding rapid steroid tapering and potent induction immunosuppression." J Hepatol 44(4): 717-722.

Bertoletti, A. and A. Gehring (2007). "Immune response and tolerance during chronic hepatitis B virus infection." Hepatol Res 37 Suppl 3: S331-338.

Bhattacharya, D. and C. L. Thio (2010). "Review of hepatitis B therapeutics." Clin Infect Dis 51(10): 1201-1208.

Blanpain, C., C. Knoop, et al. (1998). "Reactivation of hepatitis B after transplantation in patients with pre-existing anti-hepatitis B surface antigen antibodies: report on three cases and review of the literature." Transplantation 66(7): 883-886.

Blasco, A., X. Forns, et al. (2006). "Hepatic venous pressure gradient identifies patients at risk of severe hepatitis C recurrence after liver transplantation." Hepatology 43(3): 492-499.

Brown, R. S. (2005). "Hepatitis C and liver transplantation." Nature 436(7053): 973-978.

Burdick, R. A., J. L. Bragg-Gresham, et al. (2003). "Patterns of hepatitis B prevalence and seroconversion in hemodialysis units from three continents: the DOPPS." Kidney Int 63(6): 2222-2229.

Buti, M., A. Mas, et al. (2007). "Adherence to Lamivudine after an early withdrawal of hepatitis B immune globulin plays an important role in the long-term prevention of hepatitis B virus recurrence." Transplantation 84(5): 650-654.

Bzowej, N., D. R. Nelson, et al. (2011). "PHOENIX: A randomized controlled trial of peginterferon alfa-2a plus ribavirin as a prophylactic treatment after liver transplantation for hepatitis C virus." Liver Transpl 17(5): 528-538.

Calne, R. Y., D. R. Davis, et al. (1971). "Immunosuppressive effects of soluble cell membrane fractions, donor blood and serum on renal allograft survival." Minerva Chir 26(13): 703-708.

Cano, O., L. Almenar, et al. (2007). "Course of patients with chronic hepatitis C virus infection undergoing heart transplantation." Transplant Proc 39(7): 2353-2354.

Carrilho, F. J., C. R. Moraes, et al. (2004). "Hepatitis B virus infection in Haemodialysis Centres from Santa Catarina State, Southern Brazil. Predictive risk factors for infection and molecular epidemiology." BMC Public Health 4: 13.

Carrion, J. A., G. Fernandez-Varo, et al. (2010). "Serum fibrosis markers identify patients with mild and progressive hepatitis C recurrence after liver transplantation." Gastroenterology 138(1): 147-158 e141.

Carrion, J. A., M. Navasa, et al. (2006). "Transient elastography for diagnosis of advanced fibrosis and portal hypertension in patients with hepatitis C recurrence after liver transplantation." Liver Transpl 12(12): 1791-1798.

Casanovas-Taltavull, T., C. Baliellas, et al. (2007). "Preliminary results of treatment with pegylated interferon alpha 2A for chronic hepatitis C virus in kidney transplant candidates on hemodialysis." Transplant Proc 39(7): 2125-2127.

Castedal, M., M. Felldin, et al. (2005). "Preemptive therapy with pegylated interferon alpha-2b and ribavirin after liver transplantation for hepatitis C cirrhosis." Transplant Proc 37(8): 3313-3314.

CDC. (2010). "Hepatitis E." Division of Viral Hepatitis Retrieved 7/9/2011, 2011.

Chaillon, A., A. Sirinelli, et al. (2011). "Sustained virologic response with ribavirin in chronic hepatitis E virus infection in heart transplantation." J Heart Lung Transplant 30(7): 841-843.

Chalasani, N., C. Manzarbeitia, et al. (2005). "Peginterferon alfa-2a for hepatitis C after liver transplantation: two randomized, controlled trials." Hepatology 41(2): 289-298.

Charlton, M. (2007). "Approach to recurrent hepatitis C following liver transplantation." Curr Gastroenterol Rep 9(1): 23-30.

Charlton, M., K. Ruppert, et al. (2004). "Long-term results and modeling to predict outcomes in recipients with HCV infection: results of the NIDDK liver transplantation database." Liver Transpl 10(9): 1120-1130.

Charlton, M. R., A. Thompson, et al. (2011). "Interleukin-28B polymorphisms are associated with histological recurrence and treatment response following liver transplantation in patients with hepatitis C virus infection." Hepatology 53(1): 317-324.
Chen, D. S. (2009). "Hepatitis B vaccination: The key towards elimination and eradication of hepatitis B." J Hepatol 50(4): 805-816.
Chen, J., L. Yi, et al. (2010). "Hepatitis B immunoglobulins and/or lamivudine for preventing hepatitis B recurrence after liver transplantation: a systematic review." J Gastroenterol Hepatol 25(5): 872-879.
Choe, W. H., S. Y. Kwon, et al. (2008). "Tenofovir plus lamivudine as rescue therapy for adefovir-resistant chronic hepatitis B in hepatitis B e antigen-positive patients with liver cirrhosis." Liver Int 28(6): 814-820.
Chung, R. T., S. Feng, et al. (2001). "Approach to the management of allograft recipients following the detection of hepatitis B virus in the prospective organ donor." Am J Transplant 1(2): 185-191.
Coffin, C. S. and N. A. Terrault (2007). "Management of hepatitis B in liver transplant recipients." J Viral Hepat 14 Suppl 1: 37-44.
Cooreman, M. P., G. Leroux-Roels, et al. (2001). "Vaccine- and hepatitis B immune globulin-induced escape mutations of hepatitis B virus surface antigen." J Biomed Sci 8(3): 237-247.
Correa, J. R., F. D. Rocha, et al. (2003). "[Long term effect of hepatitis B and C virus infection on the survival of kidney transplant patients]." Rev Assoc Med Bras 49(4): 389-394.
Covic, A., L. Iancu, et al. (1999). "Hepatitis virus infection in haemodialysis patients from Moldavia." Nephrol Dial Transplant 14(1): 40-45.
Crippin, J. S., T. McCashland, et al. (2002). "A pilot study of the tolerability and efficacy of antiviral therapy in hepatitis C virus-infected patients awaiting liver transplantation." Liver Transpl 8(4): 350-355.
Cruzado, J. M., T. Casanovas-Taltavull, et al. (2003). "Pretransplant interferon prevents hepatitis C virus-associated glomerulonephritis in renal allografts by HCV-RNA clearance." Am J Transplant 3(3): 357-360.
Dan, Y. Y., C. T. Wai, et al. (2006). "Prophylactic strategies for hepatitis B patients undergoing liver transplant: a cost-effectiveness analysis." Liver Transpl 12(5): 736-746.
DaRoza, G., A. Loewen, et al. (2003). "Stage of chronic kidney disease predicts seroconversion after hepatitis B immunization: earlier is better." Am J Kidney Dis 42(6): 1184-1192.
Davila, S., F. E. Froeling, et al. (2010). "New genetic associations detected in a host response study to hepatitis B vaccine." Genes Immun 11(3): 232-238.
Davis, G. L., D. R. Nelson, et al. (2005). "A randomized, open-label study to evaluate the safety and pharmacokinetics of human hepatitis C immune globulin (Civacir) in liver transplant recipients." Liver Transpl 11(8): 941-949.
de Jong, Y. P., C. M. Rice, et al. (2010). "New horizons for studying human hepatotropic infections." J Clin Invest 120(3): 650-653.
de Vera, M. E., I. Dvorchik, et al. (2006). "Survival of liver transplant patients coinfected with HIV and HCV is adversely impacted by recurrent hepatitis C." Am J Transplant 6(12): 2983-2993.
Dienstag, J. L. (2008). "Hepatitis B virus infection." N Engl J Med 359(14): 1486-1500.

Dodson, S. F., M. E. de Vera, et al. (2000). "Lamivudine after hepatitis B immune globulin is effective in preventing hepatitis B recurrence after liver transplantation." Liver Transpl 6(4): 434-439.

Doucette, K. E., J. Weinkauf, et al. (2007). "Treatment of hepatitis C in potential lung transplant candidates." Transplantation 83(12): 1652-1655.

Drobeniuc, J., J. Meng, et al. (2010). "Serologic assays specific to immunoglobulin M antibodies against hepatitis E virus: pangenotypic evaluation of performances." Clin Infect Dis 51(3): e24-27.

Dulai, G., L. Higa, et al. (1999). "Successful use of lamivudine for severe acute hepatitis B virus infection in a cardiac transplant recipient." Transplantation 67(9): 1288-1289.

Dumortier, J., P. Chevallier, et al. (2003). "Combined lamivudine and hepatitis B immunoglobulin for the prevention of hepatitis B recurrence after liver transplantation: long-term results." Am J Transplant 3(8): 999-1002.

Dwyre, D. M., P. V. Holland, et al. (2008). Hepatitis viruses

Transfusion Microbiology, Cambridge University Press.

Edey, M., K. Barraclough, et al. (2010). "Review article: Hepatitis B and dialysis." Nephrology (Carlton) 15(2): 137-145.

Elamin, S. and H. Abu-Aisha (2011). "Prevention of hepatitis B virus and hepatitis C virus transmission in hemodialysis centers: review of current international recommendations." Arab J Nephrol Transplant 4(1): 35-47.

Fabrega, E., C. Garcia-Suarez, et al. (2003). "Liver transplantation with allografts from hepatitis B core antibody-positive donors: a new approach." Liver Transpl 9(9): 916-920.

Fabrizi, F., S. Bunnapradist, et al. (2005). "Treatment of hepatitis C in potential kidney and heart transplant patients." Clin Liver Dis 9(3): 487-503, viii.

Fabrizi, F., G. Lunghi, et al. (2002). "Hepatitis B virus infection in hemodialysis: recent discoveries." J Nephrol 15(5): 463-468.

Farci, P. (2003). "Delta hepatitis: an update." J Hepatol 39 Suppl 1: S212-219.

Farci, P., T. Roskams, et al. (2004). "Long-term benefit of interferon alpha therapy of chronic hepatitis D: regression of advanced hepatic fibrosis." Gastroenterology 126(7): 1740-1749.

Feray, C., A. L. Zignego, et al. (1990). "Persistent hepatitis B virus infection of mononuclear blood cells without concomitant liver infection. The liver transplantation model." Transplantation 49(6): 1155-1158.

Fishman, J. A. (2007). "Infection in solid-organ transplant recipients." N Engl J Med 357(25): 2601-2614.

Fissell, R. B., J. L. Bragg-Gresham, et al. (2004). "Patterns of hepatitis C prevalence and seroconversion in hemodialysis units from three continents: the DOPPS." Kidney Int 65(6): 2335-2342.

Forman, L. M., J. D. Lewis, et al. (2002). "The association between hepatitis C infection and survival after orthotopic liver transplantation." Gastroenterology 122(4): 889-896.

Forns, X. and J. Costa (2006). "HCV virological assessment." J Hepatol 44(1 Suppl): S35-39.

Foster, W. Q., A. Murphy, et al. (2006). "Hepatitis B vaccination in heart transplant candidates." J Heart Lung Transplant 25(1): 106-109.

Franco, E., C. Giambi, et al. (2003). "Risk groups for hepatitis A virus infection." Vaccine 21(19-20): 2224-2233.

Gane, E. J. (2008). "The natural history of recurrent hepatitis C and what influences this." Liver Transpl 14 Suppl 2: S36-44.

Gane, E. J., P. W. Angus, et al. (2007). "Lamivudine plus low-dose hepatitis B immunoglobulin to prevent recurrent hepatitis B following liver transplantation." Gastroenterology 132(3): 931-937.

Garcia-Retortillo, M., X. Forns, et al. (2004). "Hepatitis C recurrence is more severe after living donor compared to cadaveric liver transplantation." Hepatology 40(3): 699-707.

Garripoli, A., V. Di Marco, et al. (1994). "Ribavirin treatment for chronic hepatitis D: a pilot study." Liver 14(3): 154-157.

Ge, D., J. Fellay, et al. (2009). "Genetic variation in IL28B predicts hepatitis C treatment-induced viral clearance." Nature 461(7262): 399-401.

Gerolami, R., V. Moal, et al. (2008). "Chronic hepatitis E with cirrhosis in a kidney-transplant recipient." N Engl J Med 358(8): 859-860.

Gerolami, R., V. Moal, et al. (2009). "Hepatitis E virus as an emerging cause of chronic liver disease in organ transplant recipients." J Hepatol 50(3): 622-624.

Gish, R. G. and T. McCashland (2006). "Hepatitis B in liver transplant recipients." Liver Transpl 12(11 Suppl 2): S54-64.

Gurusamy, K. S., E. Tsochatzis, et al. (2010). "Antiviral prophylactic intervention for chronic hepatitis C virus in patients undergoing liver transplantation." Cochrane Database Syst Rev(12): CD006573.

Haagsma, E. B., H. G. Niesters, et al. (2009). "Prevalence of hepatitis E virus infection in liver transplant recipients." Liver Transpl 15(10): 1225-1228.

Hadziyannis, S. J., N. C. Tassopoulos, et al. (2003). "Adefovir dipivoxil for the treatment of hepatitis B e antigen-negative chronic hepatitis B." N Engl J Med 348(9): 800-807.

Hayney, M. S., D. L. Welter, et al. (2003). "High-dose hepatitis B vaccine in patients waiting for lung transplantation." Pharmacotherapy 23(5): 555-560.

Heathcote, E. J., P. Marcellin, et al. (2011). "Three-year efficacy and safety of tenofovir disoproxil fumarate treatment for chronic hepatitis B." Gastroenterology 140(1): 132-143.

Humar, A., M. Morris, et al. (2010). "Nucleic Acid Testing (NAT) of Organ Donors: Is the 'Best' Test the Right Test? A Consensus Conference Report." American Journal of Transplantation 10(4): 889-899.

Hynicka, L. M., N. Yunker, et al. (2010). "A review of oral antiretroviral therapy for the treatment of chronic hepatitis B." Ann Pharmacother 44(7-8): 1271-1286.

Jacobson, I., J. McHutchison, et al. (2010). "Telaprevir in combination with peginterferon and ribavirin in genotype 1 HCV treatment-naive patients: final results of phase 3 ADVANCE study." Hepatology 52: 427A.

Jadoul, M., J. L. Poignet, et al. (2004). "The changing epidemiology of hepatitis C virus (HCV) infection in haemodialysis: European multicentre study." Nephrol Dial Transplant 19(4): 904-909.

Jiang, L. and L. N. Yan (2010). "Current therapeutic strategies for recurrent hepatitis B virus infection after liver transplantation." World J Gastroenterol 16(20): 2468-2475.

Jimenez-Perez, M., A. B. Saez-Gomez, et al. (2010). "Efficacy and safety of entecavir and/or tenofovir for prophylaxis and treatment of hepatitis B recurrence post-liver transplant." Transplant Proc 42(8): 3167-3168.

Jungers, P., P. Devillier, et al. (1994). "Randomised placebo-controlled trial of recombinant interleukin-2 in chronic uraemic patients who are non-responders to hepatitis B vaccine." Lancet 344(8926): 856-857.

Kamar, N., A. Boulestin, et al. (2005). "Factors accelerating liver fibrosis progression in renal transplant patients receiving ribavirin monotherapy for chronic hepatitis C." J Med Virol 76(1): 61-68.

Kamar, N., C. Garrouste, et al. (2011). "Factors associated with chronic hepatitis in patients with hepatitis E virus infection who have received solid organ transplants." Gastroenterology 140(5): 1481-1489.

Kamar, N., J. M. Mansuy, et al. (2008). "Hepatitis E virus-related cirrhosis in kidney- and kidney-pancreas-transplant recipients." Am J Transplant 8(8): 1744-1748.

Kamar, N., D. Ribes, et al. (2006). "Treatment of hepatitis C virus infection (HCV) after renal transplantation: implications for HCV-positive dialysis patients awaiting a kidney transplant." Transplantation 82(7): 853-856.

Kamar, N., L. Rostaing, et al. (2010). "Pegylated interferon-alpha for treating chronic hepatitis E virus infection after liver transplantation." Clin Infect Dis 50(5): e30-33.

Kamar, N., L. Rostaing, et al. (2010). "Ribavirin therapy inhibits viral replication on patients with chronic hepatitis e virus infection." Gastroenterology 139(5): 1612-1618.

Kasiske, B. L., M. G. Zeier, et al. (2010). "KDIGO clinical practice guideline for the care of kidney transplant recipients: a summary." Kidney Int 77(4): 299-311.

Keating, G. M. and S. Noble (2003). "Recombinant hepatitis B vaccine (Engerix-B): a review of its immunogenicity and protective efficacy against hepatitis B." Drugs 63(10): 1021-1051.

Kennedy, M. and S. P. Alexopoulos (2010). "Hepatitis B virus infection and liver transplantation." Curr Opin Organ Transplant 15(3): 310-315.

Khuroo, M. S. (1980). "Study of an epidemic of non-A, non-B hepatitis. Possibility of another human hepatitis virus distinct from post-transfusion non-A, non-B type." Am J Med 68(6): 818-824.

Kim, W. R., R. H. Wiesner, et al. (1999). "Hepatic retransplantation in cholestatic liver disease: impact of the interval to retransplantation on survival and resource utilization." Hepatology 30(2): 395-400.

Klintmalm, G. B., W. K. Washburn, et al. (2007). "Corticosteroid-free immunosuppression with daclizumab in HCV(+) liver transplant recipients: 1-year interim results of the HCV-3 study." Liver Transpl 13(11): 1521-1531.

Knoll, A., M. Pietrzyk, et al. (2005). "Solid-organ transplantation in HBsAg-negative patients with antibodies to HBV core antigen: low risk of HBV reactivation." Transplantation 79(11): 1631-1633.

Ko, W. J., N. K. Chou, et al. (2001). "Hepatitis B virus infection in heart transplant recipients in a hepatitis B endemic area." J Heart Lung Transplant 20(8): 865-875.

Kornberg, A., B. Kupper, et al. (2007). "Antiviral maintenance treatment with interferon and ribavirin for recurrent hepatitis C after liver transplantation: pilot study." J Gastroenterol Hepatol 22(12): 2135-2142.

Kuo, A., J. L. Dienstag, et al. (2004). "Tenofovir disoproxil fumarate for the treatment of lamivudine-resistant hepatitis B." Clin Gastroenterol Hepatol 2(3): 266-272.

Kuo, M. Y., M. Chao, et al. (1989). "Initiation of replication of the human hepatitis delta virus genome from cloned DNA: role of delta antigen." J Virol 63(5): 1945-1950.

Lada, O., Y. Benhamou, et al. (2004). "In vitro susceptibility of lamivudine-resistant hepatitis B virus to adefovir and tenofovir." Antivir Ther 9(3): 353-363.

Lai, C. L., J. Dienstag, et al. (2003). "Prevalence and clinical correlates of YMDD variants during lamivudine therapy for patients with chronic hepatitis B." Clin Infect Dis 36(6): 687-696.

Lake, J. R. (2006). "Immunosuppression and outcomes of patients transplanted for hepatitis C." J Hepatol 44(4): 627-629.

Lauer, G. M. and B. D. Walker (2001). "Hepatitis C virus infection." N Engl J Med 345(1): 41-52.

Legrand-Abravanel, F., N. Kamar, et al. (2011). "Hepatitis E virus infection without reactivation in solid-organ transplant recipients, France." Emerg Infect Dis 17(1): 30-37.

Lerut, J. P., M. Donataccio, et al. (1999). "Liver transplantation and HBsAg-positive postnecrotic cirrhosis: adequate immunoprophylaxis and delta virus co-infection as the significant determinants of long-term prognosis." J Hepatol 30(4): 706-714.

Levitsky, J. and K. Doucette (2009). "Viral hepatitis in solid organ transplant recipients." Am J Transplant 9 Suppl 4: S116-130.

Levitsky, J., K. Thudi, et al. (2011). "Alemtuzumab induction in non-hepatitis C positive liver transplant recipients." Liver Transpl 17(1): 32-37.

Levy, G., G. L. Grazi, et al. (2006). "12-month follow-up analysis of a multicenter, randomized, prospective trial in de novo liver transplant recipients (LIS2T) comparing cyclosporine microemulsion (C2 monitoring) and tacrolimus." Liver Transpl 12(10): 1464-1472.

Lok, A. S. (2002). "Chronic hepatitis B." N Engl J Med 346(22): 1682-1683.

Lu, L., C. Li, et al. (2006). "Phylogenetic analysis of global hepatitis E virus sequences: genetic diversity, subtypes and zoonosis." Rev Med Virol 16(1): 5-36.

Lunel, F., J. F. Cadranel, et al. (2000). "Hepatitis virus infections in heart transplant recipients: epidemiology, natural history, characteristics, and impact on survival." Gastroenterology 119(4): 1064-1074.

Mallet, V., E. Nicand, et al. (2010). "Brief communication: case reports of ribavirin treatment for chronic hepatitis E." Ann Intern Med 153(2): 85-89.

Mansuy, J. M., F. Abravanel, et al. (2009). "Acute hepatitis E in south-west France over a 5-year period." J Clin Virol 44(1): 74-77.

Marcellin, P., E. J. Heathcote, et al. (2008). "Tenofovir disoproxil fumarate versus adefovir dipivoxil for chronic hepatitis B." N Engl J Med 359(23): 2442-2455.

Marcos, A., B. Eghtesad, et al. (2004). "Use of alemtuzumab and tacrolimus monotherapy for cadaveric liver transplantation: with particular reference to hepatitis C virus." Transplantation 78(7): 966-971.

Markowitz, J. S., P. Martin, et al. (1998). "Prophylaxis against hepatitis B recurrence following liver transplantation using combination lamivudine and hepatitis B immune globulin." Hepatology 28(2): 585-589.

Martin, P., R. W. Busuttil, et al. (2004). "Impact of tacrolimus versus cyclosporine in hepatitis C virus-infected liver transplant recipients on recurrent hepatitis: a prospective, randomized trial." Liver Transpl 10(10): 1258-1262.

Marzano, A., S. Gaia, et al. (2005). "Viral load at the time of liver transplantation and risk of hepatitis B virus recurrence." Liver Transpl 11(4): 402-409.

Mathurin, P., C. Mouquet, et al. (1999). "Impact of hepatitis B and C virus on kidney transplantation outcome." Hepatology 29(1): 257-263.

McAlister, V. C., E. Haddad, et al. (2006). "Cyclosporin versus tacrolimus as primary immunosuppressant after liver transplantation: a meta-analysis." Am J Transplant 6(7): 1578-1585.

McCaughan, G. W., J. Spencer, et al. (1999). "Lamivudine therapy in patients undergoing liver transplantation for hepatitis B virus precore mutant-associated infection: high resistance rates in treatment of recurrence but universal prevention if used as prophylaxis with very low dose hepatitis B immune globulin." Liver Transpl Surg 5(6): 512-519.

Mederacke, I., B. Bremer, et al. (2010). "Establishment of a novel quantitative hepatitis D virus (HDV) RNA assay using the Cobas TaqMan platform to study HDV RNA kinetics." J Clin Microbiol 48(6): 2022-2029.

Meyers, C. M., L. B. Seeff, et al. (2003). "Hepatitis C and renal disease: an update." Am J Kidney Dis 42(4): 631-657.

Montalbano, M., L. Pasulo, et al. (2007). "Treatment with pegylated interferon and ribavirin for hepatitis C virus-associated severe cryoglobulinemia in a liver/kidney transplant recipient." J Clin Gastroenterol 41(2): 216-220.

Mousa, D. H., A. H. Abdalla, et al. (2004). "Alpha-interferon with ribavirin in the treatment of hemodialysis patients with hepatitis C." Transplant Proc 36(6): 1831-1834.

Mukherjee, S. and K. Ariyarantha (2007). "Successful Hepatitis C Eradication With Preservation of Renal Function in a Liver/kidney Transplant Recipient Using Pegylated Interferon and Ribavirin." Transplantation 84(10): 1374-1375.

Nagafuchi, S., S. Kashiwagi, et al. (1991). "Reversal of nonresponders and postexposure prophylaxis by intradermal hepatitis B vaccination in Japanese medical personnel." JAMA 265(20): 2679-2683.

Navaneethan, U., M. Al Mohajer, et al. (2008). "Hepatitis E and pregnancy: understanding the pathogenesis." Liver Int 28(9): 1190-1199.

Neff, G. W., J. Nery, et al. (2004). "Tenofovir therapy for lamivudine resistance following liver transplantation." Ann Pharmacother 38(12): 1999-2004.

Neff, G. W., C. B. O'Brien, et al. (2004). "Factors that identify survival after liver retransplantation for allograft failure caused by recurrent hepatitis C infection." Liver Transpl 10(12): 1497-1503.

Nery, J. R., C. Nery-Avila, et al. (2003). "Use of liver grafts from donors positive for antihepatitis B-core antibody (anti-HBc) in the era of prophylaxis with hepatitis-B immunoglobulin and lamivudine." Transplantation 75(8): 1179-1186.

Neumann, A. U., N. P. Lam, et al. (1998). "Hepatitis C viral dynamics in vivo and the antiviral efficacy of interferon-alpha therapy." Science 282(5386): 103-107.

Neumann, U. P., T. Berg, et al. (2004). "Fibrosis progression after liver transplantation in patients with recurrent hepatitis C." J Hepatol 41(5): 830-836.

Niro, G. A., A. Ciancio, et al. (2006). "Pegylated interferon alpha-2b as monotherapy or in combination with ribavirin in chronic hepatitis delta." Hepatology 44(3): 713-720.

Niro, G. A., A. Ciancio, et al. (2005). "Lamivudine therapy in chronic delta hepatitis: a multicentre randomized-controlled pilot study." Aliment Pharmacol Ther 22(3): 227-232.

O'Grady, J. G., H. M. Smith, et al. (1992). "Hepatitis B virus reinfection after orthotopic liver transplantation. Serological and clinical implications." J Hepatol 14(1): 104-111.
Ohnishi, S., J. H. Kang, et al. (2006). "Comparison of clinical features of acute hepatitis caused by hepatitis E virus (HEV) genotypes 3 and 4 in Sapporo, Japan." Hepatol Res 36(4): 301-307.
Okuda, M., K. Hino, et al. (1999). "Differences in hypervariable region 1 quasispecies of hepatitis C virus in human serum, peripheral blood mononuclear cells, and liver." Hepatology 29(1): 217-222.
Opelz, G. and B. Dohler (2004). "Lymphomas after solid organ transplantation: a collaborative transplant study report." Am J Transplant 4(2): 222-230.
Orens, J. B., M. Estenne, et al. (2006). "International guidelines for the selection of lung transplant candidates: 2006 update--a consensus report from the Pulmonary Scientific Council of the International Society for Heart and Lung Transplantation." J Heart Lung Transplant 25(7): 745-755.
Orlowski, J., C. Alexander, et al. (2009). "Nucleic Acid Testing (NAT) for HIV, HBV, and HCV: Current Practices of 58 US Organ Procurement Organizations (OPOs)." Am J Transplant 9(Suppl 2): 555.
Ottobrelli, A., A. Marzano, et al. (1991). "Patterns of hepatitis delta virus reinfection and disease in liver transplantation." Gastroenterology 101(6): 1649-1655.
Papatheodoridis, G. V., S. Manolakopoulos, et al. (2008). "Therapeutic strategies in the management of patients with chronic hepatitis B virus infection." Lancet Infect Dis 8(3): 167-178.
Park, S. K., W. S. Yang, et al. (2001). "Outcome of renal transplantation in hepatitis B surface antigen-positive patients after introduction of lamivudine." Nephrol Dial Transplant 16(11): 2222-2228.
Pascarella, S. and F. Negro (2011). "Hepatitis D virus: an update." Liver Int 31(1): 7-21.
Patterson, S. J., J. George, et al. (2011). "Tenofovir disoproxil fumarate rescue therapy following failure of both lamivudine and adefovir dipivoxil in chronic hepatitis B." Gut 60(2): 247-254.
Peek, R. and K. R. Reddy (2007). "Hepatitis C virus-infected donors in liver transplantation." Gastroenterology 133(2): 381-382.
Perrillo, R., J. Rakela, et al. (1999). "Multicenter study of lamivudine therapy for hepatitis B after liver transplantation. Lamivudine Transplant Group." Hepatology 29(5): 1581-1586.
Perrillo, R., E. Schiff, et al. (2000). "Adefovir dipivoxil for the treatment of lamivudine-resistant hepatitis B mutants." Hepatology 32(1): 129-134.
Ponzetto, A., B. H. Hoyer, et al. (1987). "Titration of the infectivity of hepatitis D virus in chimpanzees." J Infect Dis 155(1): 72-78.
Poordad, F., J. McCone, Jr., et al. (2011). "Boceprevir for untreated chronic HCV genotype 1 infection." N Engl J Med 364(13): 1195-1206.
Potthoff, A., H. L. Tillmann, et al. (2006). "Improved outcome of chronic hepatitis B after heart transplantation by long-term antiviral therapy." J Viral Hepat 13(11): 734-741.
Poynard, T. (2004). "Treatment of hepatitis C virus: the first decade." Semin Liver Dis 24 Suppl 2: 19-24.
Prakoso, E., S. I. Strasser, et al. (2006). "Long-term lamivudine monotherapy prevents development of hepatitis B virus infection in hepatitis B surface-antigen negative

liver transplant recipients from hepatitis B core-antibody-positive donors." Clin Transplant 20(3): 369-373.
Purcell, R. H. and S. U. Emerson (2008). "Hepatitis E: an emerging awareness of an old disease." J Hepatol 48(3): 494-503.
Rasmussen, A., H. F. Davies, et al. (1995). "Combined transplantation of liver and kidney from the same donor protects the kidney from rejection and improves kidney graft survival." Transplantation 59(6): 919-921.
Rasshofer, R., S. S. Choi, et al. (1991). "Interference of antiviral substances with replication of hepatitis delta virus RNA in primary woodchuck hepatocytes." Prog Clin Biol Res 364: 223-234.
Rizzetto, M., A. Ponzetto, et al. (1991). "Epidemiology of hepatitis delta virus: overview." Prog Clin Biol Res 364: 1-20.
Robertson, B., G. Myers, et al. (1998). "Classification, nomenclature, and database development for hepatitis C virus (HCV) and related viruses: proposals for standardization. International Committee on Virus Taxonomy." Arch Virol 143(12): 2493-2503.
Roche, B., C. Feray, et al. (2003). "HBV DNA persistence 10 years after liver transplantation despite successful anti-HBS passive immunoprophylaxis." Hepatology 38(1): 86-95.
Rostaing, L., J. Izopet, et al. (1995). "Treatment of chronic hepatitis C with recombinant interferon alpha in kidney transplant recipients." Transplantation 59(10): 1426-1431.
Sahi, H., N. N. Zein, et al. (2007). "Outcomes after lung transplantation in patients with chronic hepatitis C virus infection." J Heart Lung Transplant 26(5): 466-471.
Samuel, D., R. Muller, et al. (1993). "Liver transplantation in European patients with the hepatitis B surface antigen." N Engl J Med 329(25): 1842-1847.
Samuel, D., A. L. Zignego, et al. (1995). "Long-term clinical and virological outcome after liver transplantation for cirrhosis caused by chronic delta hepatitis." Hepatology 21(2): 333-339.
Sarwal, M. M., J. Benjamin, et al. (2011). "Transplantomics and biomarkers in organ transplantation: a report from the first international conference." Transplantation 91(4): 379-382.
Scherer, M. N., B. Banas, et al. (2007). "Current concepts and perspectives of immunosuppression in organ transplantation." Langenbecks Arch Surg 392(5): 511-523.
Schiff, E. R., C. L. Lai, et al. (2003). "Adefovir dipivoxil therapy for lamivudine-resistant hepatitis B in pre- and post-liver transplantation patients." Hepatology 38(6): 1419-1427.
Seehofer, D. and T. Berg (2005). "Prevention of hepatitis B recurrence after liver transplantation." Transplantation 80(1 Suppl): S120-124.
Shrestha, M. P., R. M. Scott, et al. (2007). "Safety and efficacy of a recombinant hepatitis E vaccine." N Engl J Med 356(9): 895-903.
Shu, K. H., J. L. Lan, et al. (2004). "Ultralow-dose alpha-interferon plus ribavirin for the treatment of active hepatitis C in renal transplant recipients." Transplantation 77(12): 1894-1896.
Singer, A. L., L. M. Kucirka, et al. (2008). "The high-risk donor: viral infections in solid organ transplantation." Curr Opin Organ Transplant 13(4): 400-404.

Skripenova, S., T. D. Trainer, et al. (2007). "Variability of grade and stage in simultaneous paired liver biopsies in patients with hepatitis C." J Clin Pathol 60(3): 321-324.
Steinman, T. I., B. N. Becker, et al. (2001). "Guidelines for the referral and management of patients eligible for solid organ transplantation." Transplantation 71(9): 1189-1204.
Sugawara, Y., J. Kaneko, et al. (2006). "Cyclosporin a for treatment of hepatitis C virus after liver transplantation." Transplantation 82(4): 579-580.
Tenney, D. J., R. E. Rose, et al. (2007). "Two-year assessment of entecavir resistance in Lamivudine-refractory hepatitis B virus patients reveals different clinical outcomes depending on the resistance substitutions present." Antimicrob Agents Chemother 51(3): 902-911.
Terrault, N. A., C. C. Holland, et al. (1996). "Interferon alfa for recurrent hepatitis B infection after liver transplantation." Liver Transpl Surg 2(2): 132-138.
Terrault, N. A., M. L. Shiffman, et al. (2007). "Outcomes in hepatitis C virus-infected recipients of living donor vs. deceased donor liver transplantation." Liver Transpl 13(1): 122-129.
Thompson, N. D., J. F. Perz, et al. (2009). "Nonhospital health care-associated hepatitis B and C virus transmission: United States, 1998-2008." Ann Intern Med 150(1): 33-39.
Todo, S., A. J. Demetris, et al. (1991). "Orthotopic liver transplantation for patients with hepatitis B virus-related liver disease." Hepatology 13(4): 619-626.
Toniutto, P., E. Fumo, et al. (2004). "Favourable outcome of adefovir-dipivoxil treatment in acute de novo hepatitis B after liver transplantation." Transplantation 77(3): 472-473.
van Bommel, F., B. Zollner, et al. (2006). "Tenofovir for patients with lamivudine-resistant hepatitis B virus (HBV) infection and high HBV DNA level during adefovir therapy." Hepatology 44(2): 318-325.
van Leusen, R., R. P. Adang, et al. (2008). "Pegylated interferon alfa-2a (40 kD) and ribavirin in haemodialysis patients with chronic hepatitis C." Nephrol Dial Transplant 23(2): 721-725.
Van Wagner, L. B., T. Baker, et al. (2009). "Outcomes of patients with hepatitis C undergoing simultaneous liver-kidney transplantation." J Hepatol 51(5): 874-880.
Vladutiu, D. S., A. Cosa, et al. (2000). "Infections with hepatitis B and C viruses in patients on maintenance dialysis in Romania and in former communist countries: yellow spots on a blank map?" J Viral Hepat 7(4): 313-319.
Watt, K., B. Veldt, et al. (2009). "A practical guide to the management of HCV infection following liver transplantation." Am J Transplant 9(8): 1707-1713.
Webster, A. C., L. P. Ruster, et al. (2010). "Interleukin 2 receptor antagonists for kidney transplant recipients." Cochrane Database Syst Rev(1): CD003897.
Wedemeyer, H., K. Pethig, et al. (1998). "Long-term outcome of chronic hepatitis B in heart transplant recipients." Transplantation 66(10): 1347-1353.
Wedemeyer, H. and S. Pischke (2011). "Hepatitis: Hepatitis E vaccination--is HEV 239 the breakthrough?" Nat Rev Gastroenterol Hepatol 8(1): 8-10.
Wedemeyer, H., C. Yurdaydin, et al. (2011). "Peginterferon plus adefovir versus either drug alone for hepatitis delta." N Engl J Med 364(4): 322-331.
Wiesner, R. H., J. S. Shorr, et al. (2005). "Mycophenolate mofetil combination therapy improves long-term outcomes after liver transplantation in patients with and without hepatitis C." Liver Transpl 11(7): 750-759.

Wiesner, R. H., M. Sorrell, et al. (2003). "Report of the first International Liver Transplantation Society expert panel consensus conference on liver transplantation and hepatitis C." Liver Transpl 9(11): S1-9.

Yakaryilmaz, F., O. A. Gurbuz, et al. (2006). "Prevalence of occult hepatitis B and hepatitis C virus infections in Turkish hemodialysis patients." Ren Fail 28(8): 729-735.

Yan, M. L., L. N. Yan, et al. (2006). "Intramuscular hepatitis B immune globulin combined with lamivudine in prevention of hepatitis B recurrence after liver transplantation." Hepatobiliary Pancreat Dis Int 5(3): 360-363.

Yang, H. I., S. N. Lu, et al. (2002). "Hepatitis B e antigen and the risk of hepatocellular carcinoma." N Engl J Med 347(3): 168-174.

Yao, F. Y., R. W. Osorio, et al. (1999). "Intramuscular hepatitis B immune globulin combined with lamivudine for prophylaxis against hepatitis B recurrence after liver transplantation." Liver Transpl Surg 5(6): 491-496.

Ying, C., E. De Clercq, et al. (2000). "Inhibition of the replication of the DNA polymerase M550V mutation variant of human hepatitis B virus by adefovir, tenofovir, L-FMAU, DAPD, penciclovir and lobucavir." J Viral Hepat 7(2): 161-165.

Yurdaydin, C., H. Bozkaya, et al. (2002). "Famciclovir treatment of chronic delta hepatitis." J Hepatol 37(2): 266-271.

Zekry, A., M. Gleeson, et al. (2004). "A prospective cross-over study comparing the effect of mycophenolate versus azathioprine on allograft function and viral load in liver transplant recipients with recurrent chronic HCV infection." Liver Transpl 10(1): 52-57.

Zheng, S., Y. Chen, et al. (2006). "Prevention of hepatitis B recurrence after liver transplantation using lamivudine or lamivudine combined with hepatitis B Immunoglobulin prophylaxis." Liver Transpl 12(2): 253-258.

Zhu, F. C., J. Zhang, et al. (2010). "Efficacy and safety of a recombinant hepatitis E vaccine in healthy adults: a large-scale, randomised, double-blind placebo-controlled, phase 3 trial." Lancet 376(9744): 895-902.

Zignego, A. L., M. De Carli, et al. (1995). "Hepatitis C virus infection of mononuclear cells from peripheral blood and liver infiltrates in chronically infected patients." J Med Virol 47(1): 58-64.

Zou, S., K. A. Dorsey, et al. (2010). "Prevalence, incidence, and residual risk of human immunodeficiency virus and hepatitis C virus infections among United States blood donors since the introduction of nucleic acid testing." Transfusion 50(7): 1495-1504.

Zylberberg, H., B. Nalpas, et al. (2002). "Severe evolution of chronic hepatitis C in renal transplantation: a case control study." Nephrol Dial Transplant 17(1): 129-133.

6

Hepatitis A: Clinical, Epidemiological and Molecular Characteristics

Zahid Hussain
Centre of Excellence in Biotechnology Research, King Saud University, Riyadh, Saudi Arabia

1. Introduction

Hepatitis A virus (HAV) is a member of the *Hepatovirus* genus of *Picornaviridae* family. HAV is a non-enveloped (naked), linear, single stranded RNA virus of an icosahedral symmetry measuring 27-32 nm in diameter (Feinstone, 1973). The infectious particle consists of capsid protein and RNA genome (Fig. 1). The buoyant density of the mature particle is 1.33g/cm^3 in CsCl solutions and the sedimentation coefficient is 160S in sucrose solutions (Ticehurst, 1983).

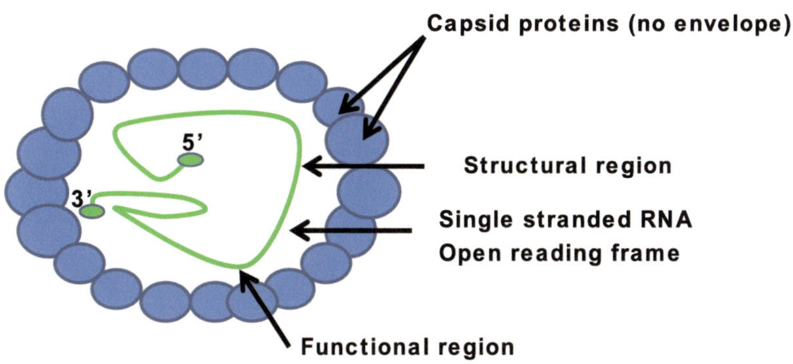

Fig. 1. The internal structure of hepatitis A virus showing capsid proteins and envelopes, structural region, single stranded RNA (open reading frame) and functional region. (Adapted from: Anderson,1988)

HAV causes an acute self limited illness. It does not lead to chronic hepatitis or a carrier state and only rarely leads to fulminant hepatic failure. HAV interferes with liver function and sparks an immune response that leads to liver inflammation (Koff, 1998). Natural infection with virus results from ingestion of fecally contaminated food and water. Virions apparently reach the liver through blood or systemic circulation and are taken up by hepatocytes (Siegl, 1988). The virus in the liver is recognized by receptor sites on the hepatocyte membrane and engulfed by the cell (Fig. 2) (Anderson, 1988). Inside the cell the virus uncoats, releases viral RNA and begins transcription (Teixeira, 1982). Once HAV completes replication in the liver, it excretes in bile and finally shed in stool.

Like all picornaviral genomes, HAV is divided into three parts: (i) 5′ non-coding region (NCR) that comprises approximately 10% of the genome (ii) single open reading frame

(ORF) of 2227 amino acids, that encode all the viral proteins, with regions designated as P1 for capsid proteins, P2 and P3 for non-structural proteins and (iii) short 3′ non-coding region (Fig. 3). HAV RNA genomes lack the cap assembly found at the 5′ end of mRNA species that normally guides the ribosomal complex to the translation start site (Najarian, 1985). Instead, an internal ribosome entry site (IRES) formed by the 5′NCR functions to initiate translations in HAV including other picornaviruses (Borman, 1997; Totsuka, 1999). However, unlike other picornavirus IRESes, the HAV IRES requires an intact eukaryotic initiation factor 4G for its optimal activity (Totsuka, 1999). Several other host proteins are found to be associated with synthetic RNAs representing segments of the 5′ NCR (Chang, 1993). The viral capsid protein (P1) is further divided into VP4, VP2, VP3 and VP1 regions. The non-structural P2 and P3 polyproteins are divided into 2A, 2B, 2C and 3A, 3B, 3C, 3D respectively (Fig. 3). HAV polyprotein is processed into precursor intermediates and mature proteins by the proteolytic activities of encoded viral proteins. HAV 2A, 2B, 2C protein encodes 45, 251 and 335 amino acids respectively. The 2A and 3C are identified as

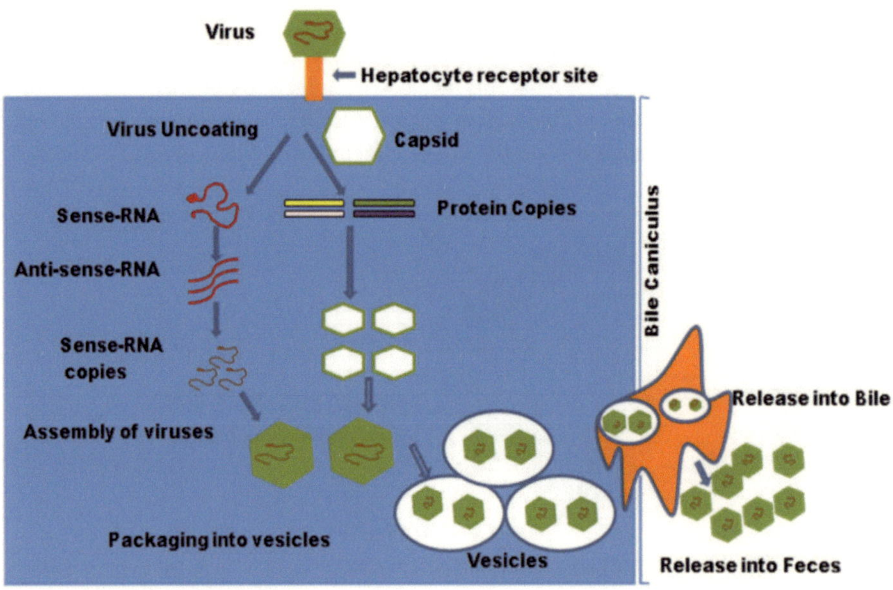

Fig. 2. Diagrammatic representation of life cycle and replicative phase of hepatitis A virus. (Adapted from: Anderson, 1988)

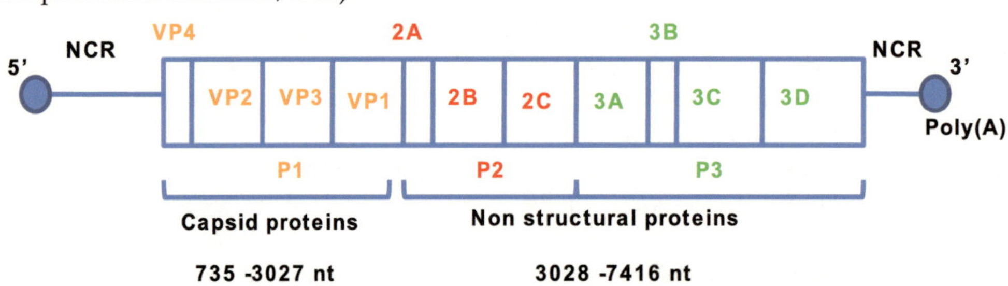

Fig. 3. Genomic structure of hepatitis A virus. HAV genome is divided into a 5′ non-coding region (5′ NCR), a giant open reading frame, and a non-coding region (3′ NCR). The coding region is subdivided into regions P1, P2 and P3. (Adapted from: Totsuka and Moritsugu, 1999)

processing enzyme in hepatitis A virus. The translated 2A regions function as intermediary, partially located on the surface (VP1) and some are assembled inside the virion (Totsuka, 1999). Both 2B and 2C proteins play an important role in the replication of the viral RNA. P3 polyproteins encodes 3A, 3B, 3C and 3D proteins with 74, 23, 219 and 489 amino acids respectively. 3C protein acts as sole protease for HAV protein processing, while 3D is the RNA dependent RNA polymerase (Schultheiss, 1994).

2. Clinical and biochemical features

Persistent infection of HAV takes four clinical phases. First phase is incubation period that varies from 15-45 days (mean 30 days) (Ciocca, 2000). HAV excretion in the faeces continued for 1-2 weeks before the onset of illness and at least 1 week afterward. The prodromal period corresponds to second phase and characterized by nonspecific symptoms followed by gastrointestinal symptoms such as nausea (loss of appetite), fatigue, abdominal pain, malaise, anorexia, fever, vomiting and flu like complaints (Lemon, 1997). These symptoms are usually short lived and followed by complete recovery. Third stage is mostly characterized by increase in bilirubin level. Jaundice becomes clinically apparent when the total bilirubin exceeds 2.0-4.0 mg/dL (Fig. 4). In half of the hepatitis A patients clinical signs such as hepatomegaly and hepatic tenderness are prominent. The final phase is a convalescent period during which the patient recovers. Signs and symptoms usually lasts for less than 2 months, although 10-15 percent of symptomatic persons have prolonged or relapsing illness lasting up to 6 months (Hussain, 2005). The increase of serum aminotransferases, bilirubin (both total and direct), and alkaline phosphatase is the most striking laboratory findings of hepatitis A. In most of the hepatitis A cases level of serum aminotransferases increases mildly, but in severe cases it may be elevated to significantly high level that ranges from 1,000-1,500 IU/liter (Hussain, 2005).

2.1 Diagnostic features

Hepatitis A cannot be differentiated from other types of viral hepatitis on the basis of clinical or epidemiologic features alone. Diagnosis of acute hepatitis A is based upon the detection of anti-HAV IgM antibodies or presence of HAV RNA in serum or faeces. In the majority of persons, serum anti-HAV IgM becomes detectable 5-10 days before onset of symptoms. IgM antibodies are detectable soon after infection and can remain detectable for about 6 months (Fig. 4). The anti-HAV IgG appears early in the course of infection and remain detectable for the person's lifetime and provides lifelong protection against the disease. Total anti-HAV testing is used in epidemiologic studies to measure the prevalence of previous infection or by clinicians to determine whether a person with an indication for pre-exposure prophylaxis is already immune. HAV RNA can be detected in the blood and stool of the majority of persons during the acute phase of infection by using nucleic acid amplification methods, and sequencing is used to determine the relatedness of HAV isolates for epidemiologic investigations. HAV RNA can also be detected in blood during the incubation period, acute phase, and 18-30 days after the onset of illness (Kwon, 2000; Hussain, 2006). However recent study suggests presence of HAV RNA for an average of 95 days and viremia persisted longer after the onsets of symptoms (average, 79 days) (Bower, 2000; Normann, 2004).

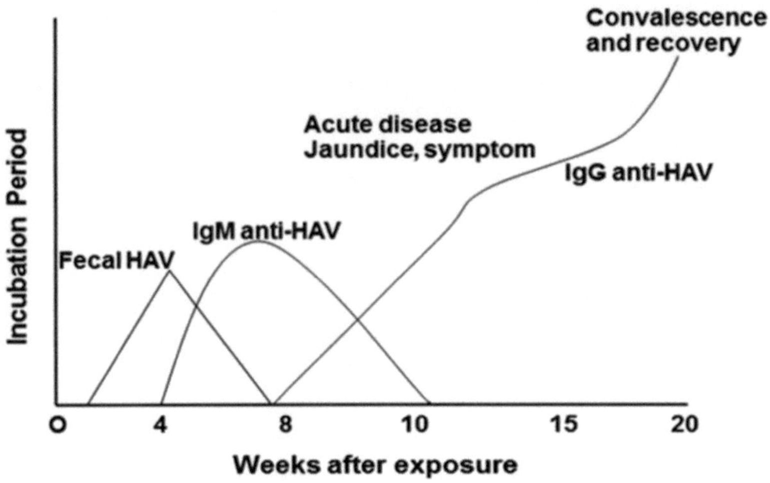

Fig. 4. The serological course of hepatitis A virus. The virus can be detected in the feces up to 2 weeks before the appearance of the jaundice and up to 2 weeks afterwards. (Adapted from Lemon, 1997)

3. Epidemiological characteristics

Hepatitis A is an enterically transmitted viral infection of public health problem all over the world. Faecally contaminated food and water is the common source of HAV infection. Consumption of contaminated food is a leading cause of large number of outbreaks in the past that affect hundreds and thousands of people (Koff, 1998). The source of most reported foodborne hepatitis A outbreaks has been HAV-infected food handlers. Waterborne transmission predominates in developing countries and is responsible for infection at early age. Therefore, it is responsible for endemicity rather than clinical outbreaks. In contrast, waterborne transmission in developed countries accounts for a very small proportion of HAV infections. Ninety percent of infections in children are subclinical or asymptomatic whereas exposure of adults and adolescents mainly leads to clinical form. Asymptomatic or unrecognized infections in children play an important role in HAV transmission and serve as a primary source of infections to others. The special groups of adult population such as men who have sex with men (MSM) or intravenous drug users (IVDUs) sustained the risk of HAV infection (Cotter, 2003; Vong, 2005). The blood borne transmission is also responsible for number of outbreaks of hepatitis A (Peerlinck, 1998; Ridolfo, 2000).

HAV Infection is hyperendemic in vast areas of the world, with approximately 1.5 million clinical cases per year (Fig. 5) (WHO, 2000). The worldwide distribution is uneven and is based on determinants such as socioeconomic conditions and geographic factors (Craig, 2004; Wasley, 2006; Jacobsen, 2010). In developing countries, the incidence of disease in adults is relatively low because of exposure to the virus in childhood. Most adults in these areas show prevalence of antibodies against hepatitis A. In developed world endemicity is usually very low and clinical cases occur almost exclusively in adults (Feinstone, 1996; Marinho, 1997). The variable age distribution among hepatitis A patients in developing and developed countries is a consequence of differing standards of hygiene and sanitation. In many developing countries, improved hygiene standards and socio-economic conditions have led to a reduction in exposure to HAV in childhood and hence large non-immune adult population in the community. This leads to a shift or transition from asymptomatic childhood infections to an increased incidence of symptomatic or clinical disease in adults (Hussain, 2006). The persistence of circulating HAV may lead to hepatitis A outbreaks in susceptible non-immune adult population (Arankalle, 2001; Hussain, 2006).

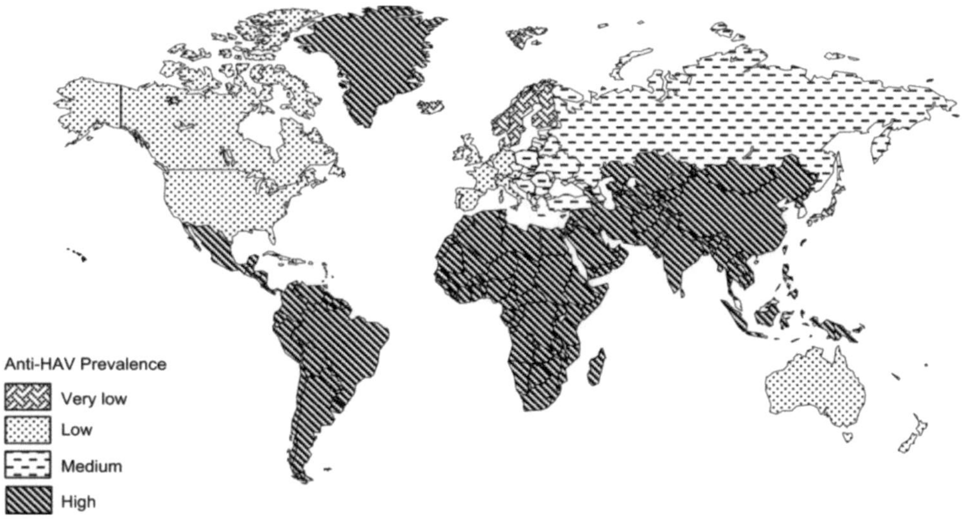

Fig. 5. The global prevalence of hepatitis A virus infection based on presence of anti-bodies to hepatitis A virus i.e. anti-HAV. (Adapted from: Wasley, 2006)

4. Molecular epidemiological characteristics

Genetic heterogeneity of hepatitis A has been revealed by sequencing different genome regions, including VP3 carboxyl terminus, the VP1 amino terminus and the VP1/2A junction (Cohen, 1987; Arauz-Ruiz, 2001; Costa-Mattioli, 2002) (fig. 6). The VP3 C-terminal region is relatively conserved, the VP1 amino acid terminus presents an intermediate variability, while VP1/2A junction is more variable and is used to distinguish one strain from another (Costa-Mattioli, 2002). The genetic variability observed within the putative VP1/2A junction (168 nucleotides) initially defined seven (I-VII) genotypes (Khanna, 1992; Robertson, 1992; Ching, 2002). However, recently new classification of HAV has been done based on the complete sequences of the 900 nucleotides of VP1 region (Costa-Mattioli, 2002) (Fig. 6). The phylogenetic analyses of VP1 sequences identified six genotypes (I-VI) that differ among themselves 15-25%. Three isolated from humans (I-III) and three from a simian origin (IV-VI). The genotypes I, II and III were further subdivided into subgenotypes A and B, which differ in approximately 7.5% of base positions.

The worldwide genotype distribution showed genotype I and III comprise the vast majority of human strains within the studied population (Fig. 7). Sub-genotype IA comprises the majority of the human strains studied and constitutes major virus population in North and South America, China, Japan, Russia and Thailand. The sub-genotype IB contains strains from Jordan, North Africa, Australia, Europe, Japan and South America. Most of the remaining human HAV strains segregate into genotype III that is further divided into two sub-genotypes, IIIA, and IIIB (Cohen, 1987; Jansen, 1990; Robertson, 1992). The sub-genotype IIIA have been subsequently identified in specimens collected from humans with hepatitis A in India, Sri

Lanka, Nepal, Malaysia, Sweden and the U.S.A [Khanna, 1992, Hussain, 2005]. The IIIB sub-genotype is responsible for cases of HAV infection in Japan and Denmark.

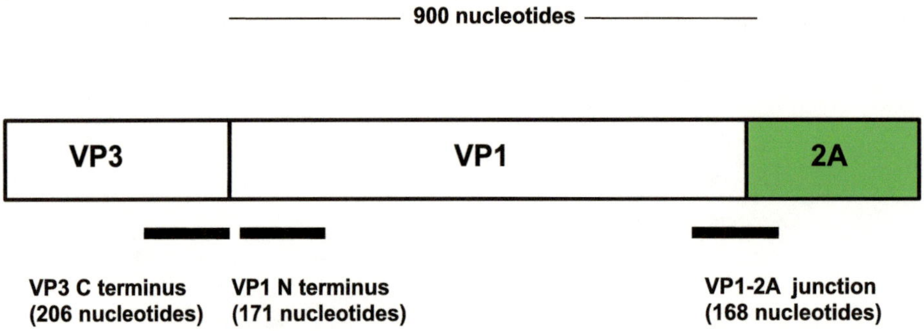

Fig. 6. The genomic organization of VP3 C-terminal, the VP1 amino acid terminal and VP1/2A junction region of hepatitis A virus. The complete sequence of the 900 nucleotides of the VP1 gene has been used for new classification of HAV. (Adapted from: Costa-Mattioli, 2003)

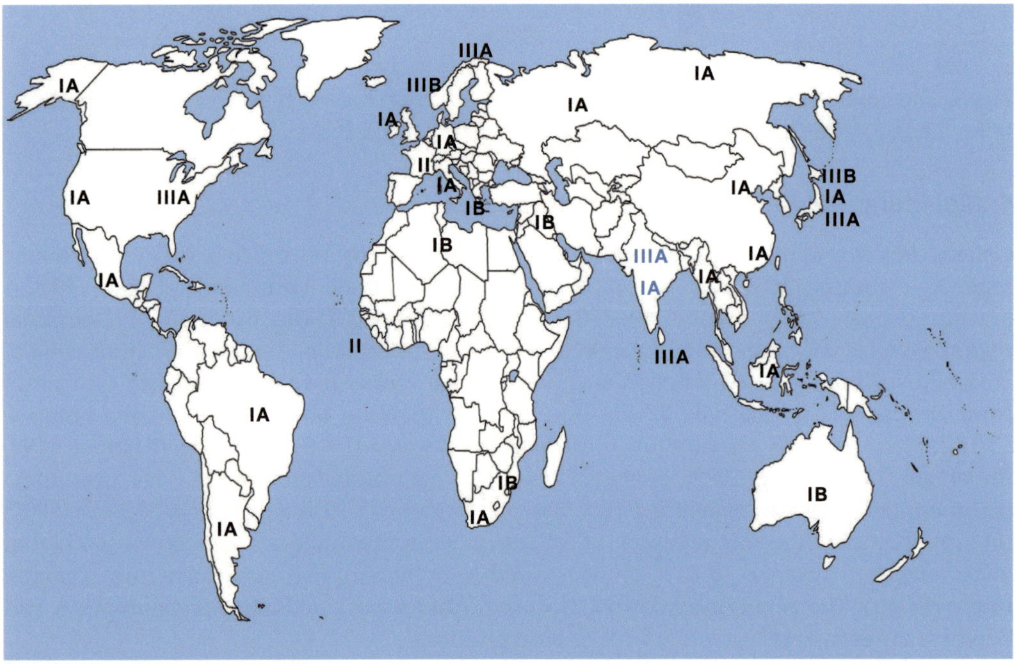

Fig. 7. Worldwide distribution of hepatitis A virus genotype(s) according to the VP3 carboxyl terminus, the VP1 amino terminus and the VP1/P2A junction. (Adapted from: Wasley, 2006)

In contrast, genotype II has rarely been reported worldwide. Recently, former genotype VII (SLF 88 isolate) has been reclassified within the genotype IIB (Costa-Mattioli, 2002; Lu, 2004) (Fig. 8 & 9). Similarly, sub-genotype II (CF-53/Berne isolate) has been defined as IIA in new HAV classification (Fig. 8 & 9).

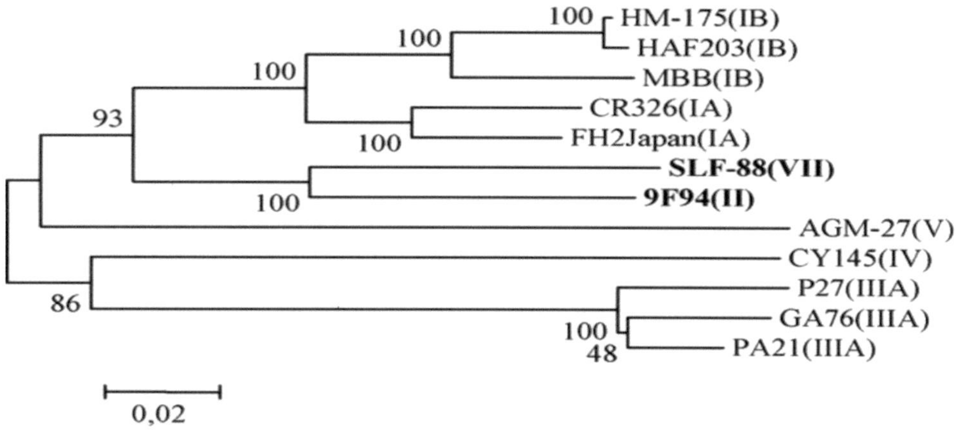

Fig. 8. Neighbour joining phylogenetic tree of the VP1/P2A region using the two-parameter model of Kimura. Genotypes and sub-genotypes are shown along with strains name. The strains (SLF-88 and 9F94) in bold has close genetic relationship and hence in latest nomenclature genotype VII has been reclassified in genotype IIB. (Adapted from: Costa-Mattioli, 2002)

The three simians genotypes were defined by unique nucleotide sequences from the P1 regions of HAV strains. In addition, all simian HAVs have a distinct signature sequence at the VP3/VP1 junction which distinguishes these strains from human HAVs.

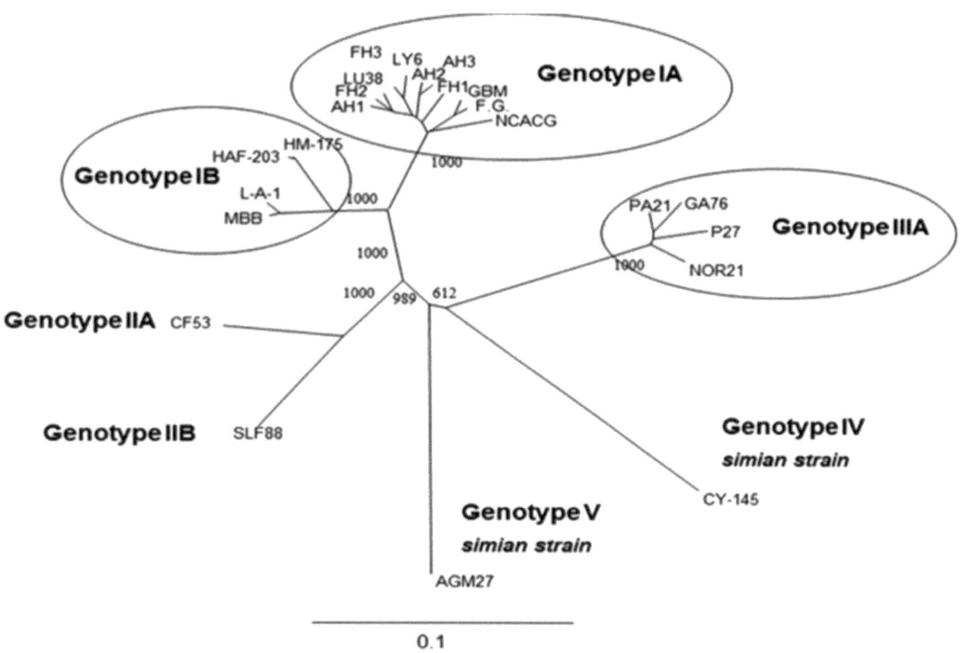

Fig. 9. The phylogenetic tree based upon the nucleotide sequence of the structural proteins showing 3 different genotypes of human isolates and 2 simian isolates. (Adapted from: Costa-Mattioli, 2002)

4.1 Application of molecular technique in deciphering outbreaks

Molecular techniques provide an important tool in decoding the epidemiological outbreaks of hepatitis A. These techniques have been successfully applied for the detection numerous HAV outbreaks linked to various sources such as clinical specimens and environmental samples such as faecally contaminated water, food (Hutin, 1999). There are several examples where molecular techniques such as RT-PCR and sequencing have been used effectively in outbreaks to definitely relate the source of infection (De Serres, 1999; Sanchez, 2002; Chironna, 2004; Arankalle, 2006; Tallon, 2008). The molecular epidemiological techniques also helped to report several outbreaks in major European cities among men who have sex with men (MSM) (Reintjes, 1999; Bell, 2001; Stene-Johansen, 2002) as well as in intravenous drug users (IVDUs) (Davidkin, 2007).

4.2 Mode of evolution in HAV

HAV replicates as complex dynamic mutant distributions and quasispecies. The evolutionary study of HAV over time also suggests continuous generation of variants or quasispecies that coexist in time and in different environment (Costa-Mattioli, 2003; Sanchez, 2003a). These findings suggest that beyond mutations and genetic recombination, HAV exploits variation strategy in dominance to promote and ensure its survival. Despite some degree of nucleotide heterogeneity at the capsid region of HAV, there is not an equivalent degree of amino acid variation (Aragonès, 2008; Pérez-Sautu, 2011). Severe structural constraints in the hepatitis A virus capsid prevent more extensive substitutions necessary for the emergence of new serotype, and hence existence of single serotype of human HAV (Bosch, 1998).

5. Complications related to hepatitis A

Fulminant hepatitis A is a rare complication, with reported incidence of 0.015 to 0.9% of overall cases worldwide (O'Gardy, 1993). The fulminant hepatitis A is occasional phenomenon during which more expensive necrosis of the liver occurs that follows impairment of hepatic synthetic processes, excretory functions and detoxifying mechanism. It occurs during the first 4-6 weeks of illness which is characterized by sudden onset of high fever, marked abdominal pain, vomiting and jaundice followed by development of hepatic encephalopathy associated with deep coma and seizures (O'Gardy, 1989; Takahashi, 1991). Mortality is highly correlated with increasing age, survival being rare over the age 45 years (Acharya, 1996). Clinical signs indicating liver failure include a rapid decrease in size of the liver, prolongation of the prothrombin time and decrease in the aminotransferase level as the bilirubin level continues to rise (Evangelos, 1989; Vento, 1998).

5.1 Mortality rate

The vast majority of hepatitis A patients make a full recovery and fatality rate is low. The estimated mortality rate is 0.1% for children less than 15 years old, 0.3% for adults ages 15 to 39, and 2.1% for adults ages 40 and old (Hollinger, 1996; Debray, 1997). The acute HAV super infection with chronic liver disease is also associated with severity and high mortality (Keffe, 1995; Vento, 1998).

5.2 Treatment

Specific treatment is not available for acute hepatitis A virus infection. As in most cases the infection is self-limiting and is followed by complete recovery without chronic sequelae, and no specific interventions are required. Patients with hepatic failure are highly recommended to transfer to centre capable of performing liver transplants.

6. HAV control and prevention strategies

HAV control and prevention strategies vary, depending on the country. The current WHO position paper (2000) includes specific positions for countries, depending on their HAV endemicity. In **highly endemic countries**, almost all persons are asymptomatically infected with HAV in childhood, which effectively prevents clinical hepatitis A in adolescents and adults. In these countries, large-scale vaccination program are not recommended. In **countries of intermediate endemicity** where a relatively large proportion of the adult population is susceptible to HAV, and where hepatitis A represents a significant public health burden, large-scale childhood vaccination may be considered as a supplement to health education and improved sanitation. In **regions of low endemicity**, vaccination against hepatitis A is indicated for individuals with increased risk of contracting the infection, such as travelers to areas of intermediate or high endemicity. Other high-risk persons include MSM and IVDUs communities (Francis, 1984; Widell, 1983). Persons with underlying chronic liver disease from any cause, particularly if they are older than 45-50, are at increased risk of fulminant hepatitis A and should be immunized. Immunization of foodhandlers could prevent common source outbreaks of hepatitis, but the cost effectiveness of such a strategy is not known (Lemon and Shapiro, 1994).

6.1 Vaccine and immune response

HAV vaccines from various manufacturers are widely available in the market throughout the world. These vaccines have tremendous response with observed anti-antibody among children (**91-100%**) and young healthy adults (**96%**) which persists for up to 15-20 years after completion of vaccination schedule (WHO, 2000; Hammitt, 2008).

7. Conclusion

HAV remain an important cause of hepatitis outbreak and is a major public health problem worldwide especially in developing countries. It is mostly reported from poor sanitary and unhygienic surroundings, which emphasizes the need for improving the public health measures to prevent epidemics of hepatitis A. The changes in epidemiological pattern would increase the disease burden, may cause large community outbreaks and lead to increased healthcare cost. The emergence of new serotype is highly unlikely, although new variants can emerge if virus population is forced to severe immune selective pressure. Since hepatitis A exists as a single serotype and human is the only host, it is possible to eradicate by selective vaccination against individuals who are susceptible and sero-negative for HAV-IgM.

8. Acknowledgments

The author extends his appreciation to the Deanship of Scientific Research at King Saud University for funding the work through the research group project number: RGP-VPP-136. He also expresses his gratitude to the Centre of Excellence in Biotechnology Research, King Saud University, Saudi Arabia, and to the staff of PCR Hepatitis Laboratory, Maulana Azad Medical College, New Delhi, India, for generous support.

9. References

Feinstone, S, M.; Kapikian, A, Z., Purcell, R, H. (1973). Hepatitis A: detection by immune electron microscopy of a virus like antigen associated with acute illness. *Science,* 182, 1026

Ticehurst J, R.; Racaniello V, R., Baroudy B, M., Baltimore, D., Purcell, R,H., Feinstone, S, M. (1983). Molecular cloning and characterization of hepatitis A virus cDNA. *Proc Natl Acad Sci* USA 80, 5885-5889

Koff, R, S. (1998). Hepatitis A. *Lancet* 351, 1643-1649

Siegl, G. (1988). Virology of hepatitis A. In: Zuckerman AJ, ed. *Viral Hepatitis and liver disease.* New York: Alan R Liss, 3-7

Anderson, D,A., Locarnini, S, A., Gust, I, D. (1988). Replication of hepatitis A virus. In: Zuckerman AJ, ed. *Viral hepatitis and liver disease,* New York: Alan R Liss, 8-11

Teixeira, M, R., Weller, I, V, D., Murray, A., et al. (1982). The pathology of hepatitis A in man. *Liver* 2, 53-60

Najarian, R., Caput, D., Gee, W., *et al.* (1985). Primary structure and gene organization of human hepatitis A virus. *Proc. Natl. Acad. Sci. USA 82,* 2627–2631

Borman, A, M., Kean, K, M. (1997). Intact eukaryotic initiation factor 4G is required for hepatitis A virus internal initiation of translation. *Virology 237,* 129–136

Totsuka, A., Moritsugu, Y. (1999). Hepatitis A virus proteins. *Intervirology 42,* 63–68

Chang, K, H., Brown, E, A., Lemon, S, M. (1993). Cell type specific proteins which interact with the 5) non translated region of hepatitis A virus RNA. *J Virol* 67, 6716–6725.

Schultheiss, T., Kusov, Y, Y., Gauss-Muller V. (1994). Proteinase 3C of hepatitis A virus (HAV) cleaves the HAV polyprotein P2-P3 at all sites including VP1/2A and 2A/2B. *Virology 198,* 275–281

Ciocca, M. (20000. Clinical course and consequences of hepatitis A infection. *Vaccine 18,* S71-74.

Lemon, S, M. (1997). Type A viral hepatitis: epidemiology, diagnosis, and prevention. *Clin Chem 43,* 1494–1499

Hussain, Z., Das, B, C., Husain, S, A., Asim, M., Chattopadhyay, S., Malik, A., Poovorawan, Y., Theamboonlers, A., Kar, P. (2005). Hepatitis A viral genotypes and clinical relevance: Clinical and molecular characterization of hepatitis A virus isolates from northern India. *Hepatol Res 32,* 16–24

Kwon, O,S., Byun, K,S., Yeon, J,E., Park, S,H., Kim, J,S., Kim, J,H., Bak, Y,T., Kim, J,H., Lee, C,H. (2000). Detection of hepatitis A viral RNA in sera of patients with acute hepatitis A. *J Gastroenterol Hepatol 15,* 1043-1047.

Hussain, Z., Das, B, C., Husain, S, A., Polipalli, S,K., Ahmed, T., Begum, N., Medhi, S., Verghese, A., Raish, M., Theamboonlers, A., Poovorawan, Y., Kar, P. (2006). Virological course of hepatitis A virus as determined by real time RT-PCR: Correlation with biochemical, immunological and genotypic profiles. *World J Gastroenterol 12*,4683-4688.

Bower, W,A., Nainan, O,V., Han, X., Margolis, H,S.(2000). Duration of viremia in hepatitis A virus infection. *J Infect Dis 18*, 12-17.

Normann, A., Jung ,C., Vallbracht, A., Flehmig, B. (2004). Time course of hepatitis A viremia and viral load in the blood of human hepatitis A patients. *J Med Virol* 72, 10-16.

Cotter S, M, Sansom, S, Long, T, et al. (2003). Outbreak of hepatitis A among men who have sex with men: implications for hepatitis A vaccination strategies. *J Infect Dis* 187,1235–1240.

Vong, S, Fiore, A, E, Haight, D, O, et al. (2005). Vaccination in the county jail as a strategy to reach high risk adults during a community-based hepatitis A outbreak among methamphetamine drug users. *Vaccine 23*, 1021–1028.

Peerlinck, K., Vermylen, J. (1993). Acute hepatitis A in patients with hemophilia A. *Lancet* 341, 179

Ridolfo, A, L., Rusconi, S., Antimori, S., Balotta, C., Galli, M. (2000). Persisting HIV-1 replication triggered by acute hepatitis A virus infection. *Antiviral Ther* 5, 15-18

World Health Organization. (2000). Hepatitis A vaccines. *Wkly Epidemiol Rec* 75, 38–44

Craig, A, S., Schaffner, W. (2004). Prevention of hepatitis A with the hepatitis A vaccine. *N Engl J Med 350*, 476-481

Wasley, A., Fiore, A., Bell, B, P. (2006). Hepatitis A in the era of vaccination. *Epidemiol Rev. 28*, 101-111

Jacobsen, K, H., Wiersma, S, T. (2010). Hepatitis A virus seroprevalence by age and world region, 1990 and 2005. *Vaccine 28*, 6653–6657

Feinstone, S, M. (1996). Hepatitis A: epidemiology and prevention. *Eur J Gastroenterol Hepatol* 8, 300-5

Marinho, R, T., Valente, A, R., Ramalho, F,J., de Moura, M, C. (1997). The changing epidemiological pattern of hepatitis A in Lisbon, Portugal. *Eur J Gastroenterol Hepatol* 9, 795-797

Hussain, Z., Das, B, C., Husain, S, A., Murthy, N, S., Kar, P. (2006). Increasing trend of acute hepatitis A in north India: need for identification of high-risk population for vaccination. *J Gastroenterol Hepatol 21*, 689–693

Arankalle, V, A., Chadha, M, S., Chitambar, S, D., Walimbe, A, M., Chobe, L, P., Gandhe, S, S. (2001). Changing epidemiology of hepatitis A and E in urban and rural India (1982–1998). *J Viral Hepat 8*, 293–303

Cohen JI, Ticehurst JR, Purcell RH, Buckler-White A, Baroudy BM. (1987). Complete nucleotide sequence of wild type hepatitis A virus: comparision with different strains of hepatitis A virus and other picornaviruses. *J Virol 61*, 50-59.

Arauz-Ruiz, P., L. Sundqvist, Z. Garcia, L. Taylor, K. Visona, H. Norder, and L. O. Magnius. (2001). Presumed common source outbreaks of hepatitis A in an endemic area confirmed by limited sequencing within the VP1 region. *J Med Virol 65*, 449–456.

Costa-Mattioli M, Cristina J, Romero H, Perez-Bercof R, Casane D, Colina R, Garcia L, Vega I, Glikman G, Romanowsky V, Castello A, Nicand E, Gassin M, Billaudel S, Ferré V. (2002). Molecular evolution of hepatitis A virus: a new classification based on the complete VP1 protein. *J Virol 76*, 9516-9525.

Khanna B, Spelbring JE, Innis BL, Robertson BH. (1992). Characterization of a genetic variant of human hepatitis A virus. *J Med Virol 36*, 118-124.

Robertson BH, Jansen RW, Khanna B *et al.* (1992). Genetic relatedness of hepatitis A virus strains recovered from different geographical regions. *J Gen Virol 73*, 1365-1377.

Ching KZ, Nakano T, Chapman LE, Demby A, Robertson BH. (2002). Genetic characterization of wild-type genotype VII hepatitis A virus. *J Gen Virol 83*, 53-60.

Jansen, R. W., G. Siegl, and S. M. Lemon. (1990). Molecular epidemiology of human hepatitis A virus defined by an antigen-capture polymerase chain reaction method. *Proc. Natl. Acad. Sci. USA 87*, 2867–2871.

Lu, L., Ching, K.Z., de Paula, V. S., Nakano, T., Siegl, G., Weitz, M., Robertson, B.H. (2004) Characterization of the complete genomic sequence of genotype II hepatitis A virus (CF53/Berne isolate). *J Gen Virol 85*, 2943–2952

Hutin, Y. J., et al., (1999). A multistate, foodborne outbreak of hepatitis A. *N Engl J Med 340*, 595-602

De Serres, G., et al., (1999) Molecular confirmation of hepatitis A virus from well water: Epidemiology and public health implications. *J Infect Dis*, *179*, 37-43

Sanchez, G., et al., (2002). Molecular characterization of hepatitis A virus isolates from a transcontinental shellfish-borne outbreak. *J Clin Microbiol 40* 4148-4155

Chironna, M., et al., (2004). Outbreak of infection with hepatitis A virus (HAV) associated with a foodhandler and confirmed by sequence analysis reveals a new HAV genotype IB variant, *J Clin Microbiol 42*, 2825-2828

Arankalle, V.A., Sarada Devi, K.L., Lole, K.S., Shenoy, K,T., Verma, V., Haneephabi, M. (2006). Molecular characterization of hepatitis A virus from a large outbreak from Kerala, India. *Indian J Med Res 123*, 760-769.

Tallon, L. A., et al., (2008). Recovery and sequence analysis of hepatitis A virus from springwater implicated in an outbreak of acute viral hepatitis, *Appl Environ Microbiol 74*, 6158-6160.

Reintjes, R., Bosman, A. de ZO., Stevens, M, van der K,L., van den, H,K. (1999). Outbreak of hepatitis A in Rotterdam associated with visits to 'darkrooms' in gay bars. *Commun Dis Public Health 2*, 43-46.

Bell, A., Ncube, F., Hansell, A., Davison, K,L., Young, Y., Gilson, R., et al. (2001). An outbreak of hepatitis A among young men associated with having sex in public venues. *Commun Dis Public Health 4*, 163-170.

Stene-Johansen, K., Jenum, P,A., Hoel, T., Blystad, H., Sunde, H., Skaug, K. (2002). An outbreak of hepatitis A among homosexuals linked to a family outbreak. *Epidemiol Infect 129*, 113-117.

Davidkin, I., Zheleznova, N., Jokinen, S., Gorchakova, O., Broman, M. and Mukomolov, S. (2007). Molecular epidemiology of hepatitis A in St. Petersburg, Russia, 1997–2003. *J Med Virol 79*, 657–662.

Costa-Mattioli, M., Di Napoli, A., Ferre, V., Billaudel, S., Perez-Bercoff, R., Cristina, J. (2003). Genetic variability of hepatitis A virus. *J Gen Virol 84*, 3191-3201

Sanchez, G., Bosch, A., Gomez-Mariano, G., Domingo, E., Pinto, R, M. (2003a). Evidence for quasispecies distributions in the human hepatitis A virus genome. *Virology 315*, 34–42

Aragonès, L., Bosch, A., Pintó, R.M. (2008). Hepatitis A virus mutant spectra under the selective pressure of monoclonal antibodies: codon usage constraints limit capsid variability. *J Virol 82*, 1688–1700.

Pérez-Sautu, U., Costafreda, M.I., Caylà, J., Tortajada, C., Lite J., Bosch, A., *et al.* (2011). Hepatitis A virus vaccine escape variants and potential new serotype emergence. *Emerg Infect Dis 17*, 734–737

Bosch, A., Gonzalez-Dankaart, J, F., Haro, I., Gajardo, R., Pe´rez, J, A., Pinto,´ R, M. (1998). A new continuous epitope of hepatitis A virus. *J Med Virol 54*, 95–102

O'Grady, J, G., Schalm, S,W., Williams, R. (1993). Acute liver failure: redefining the syndromes. *Lancet, 342*, 273-275

Takashaki, Y., Okuda, K. (1993). Fulminant and subfulminant hepatitis in Japan. *Indian J Gastroenterol 12*, 19-21

Acharya, S, K., Dasarathy, S., Kumer, T,L., Sushma, S., Prasanna, K,S., Tandon, A., Sreenivas, V., Nijhawan, S., Panda, S, K., Nanda, S, K., Irshad, M., Joshi, Y, K., Duttagupta, S., Tandon, R, K., Tandon, B, N. (1996). Fulminant hepatitis in a tropical population: clinical course, cause, and early predictors of outcome. *Hepatology*, 23, 1448-1455

Evangelos, A., Akriviadis, E, A., Redker, A, G. (1989). Fulminant hepatitis A in intravenous drug users with chronic liver disease. *Ann Intern Med 110*, 838

Vento, S., Garofano, T., Rezzini, C., Cainelli, F., Casali, F., Ghirozi, G., Ferraro, T., Concai, E. (1998). Fulminant hepatitis associated with hepatitis A virus superinfection in patients with chronic C. *N Engl J Med* , 29, 286-290

Hollinger, F.B., Ticehurst, J,R. (1996). Hepatitis A virus. *Fields Virology*, 3rd ed.; Fields, B.N., Knipe, D.M., Howley, O.M., *et al.* Eds.; Lippincott Williams & Wilkins: Philadelphia, NY, USA, pp. 735–782.

Debray, D., Cullufi, P., Devictor, D., Fabre, M., Bernard, O. (1997). Liver failure in children with hepatitis A. *Hepatology* 26, 1018-1022.

Keeffe, E,B. (1995). Is hepatitis A more severe in patients with chronic hepatitis B and other chronic liver disease? *Am J Gastroenterol* 90, 201-205.

Francis, D,P., Hadler, S,C., Prendergast, T,J., Peterson, E., Ginsberg, M, M. Lookabaugh, C., et al. (1984). Occurrence of hepatitis A, B, and non-A/ non-B in the United States. CDC sentinel county hepatitis study I. Am J Med ,76, 69–74.

Widell, A., Hansson, B, G., Moestrup, T., Nordenfelt, E. (1983). Increased occurrence of hepatitis A with cyclic outbreaks among drug addicts in a Swedish community. *Infection* 11, 198–200.

Lemon, S,M., Shapiro, C,N. (1994). The value of immunization against hepatitis A. Infect Agents Dis , 3, 38–49.

Hammitt, L,L., Bulkow, L., Hennessy, T,W., Zanis, C., Snowball, M., Williams, J,L., Bell, B,P., McMahon, B,J. (2008). Persistence of antibody to hepatitis A virus 10 years after vaccination among children and adults. *J Infect Dis 198*, 1776-1782.

7

Structure and Function of the Hepatitis E Virus Capsid Related to Hepatitis E Pathogenesis

Zheng Liu[1], Yizhi Jane Tao[2] and Jingqiang Zhang[1]
[1]*State Key Laboratory for Biocontrol, Sun Yat-Sen University, Guangzhou,*
[2]*Department of Biochemistry and Cell Biology, Rice University, Houston, TX*
China
USA

1. Introduction

There are five different types of viral hepatitis (A, B, C, D, and E) in the world, each of which caused by a different virus. Although they all cause the disease in human, the five viruses are unrelated and are from different virus families with totally different genome structures and distinct replication mechanisms (Fauquet et al., 2005; Hochman & Balistreri, 1999; Kumar et al., 2010). Hepatitis E is an acute viral hepatitis caused by hepatitis E virus (HEV) which is transmitted primarily through a fecal-oral route (Knipe et al., 2007). Pregnancy is one of the risk factors for severe HEV infection with high mortality rate. Numerous epidemic and sporadic cases have occurred in developing countries of Asia, the Middle East, and North Africa, where sanitary conditions are not well-maintained (Okamoto, 2007; Panda et al., 2007; Vasickova et al., 2007). Recent epidemiological studies show that significant prevalence of HEV and anti-HEV antibody is found in humans and several kinds of wild and domestic animals worldwide, including industrialized countries (Meng, 2010).

Hepatitis E virus, discovered in 1983 by immune electron microscopy (Balayan et al., 1983) and first cloned in 1990 (Reyes et al., 1990), is the sole member of the genus Hepevirus within the family Hepeviridae. Based on genome sequences, five major genotypes have been identified. The circulation of genotypes 1 and 2 viruses is maintained among only humans, while those of genotypes 3 and 4 are found in human as well as animals. The viruses of genotype 5 are of avian origin, thought to be noninfectious to humans. Although four of the five genotypes infect human ,only one HEV serotype has been found in human (Okamoto, 2007).

HEV is composed of a protein capsid made of a single protein and a positive-sense RNA genome of 7.2 to 7.8 kb in size. Like the hepatitis A virus (HAV), HEV does not have a viral envelope, different from the hepatitis B, C, D virus, all of which contain membrane envelopes outside their capsid. The genomic RNA of HEV is capped, polyadenylated, containing three open reading frames (ORFs). ORF1, mapped at the 5′ terminus of the genome, has about 5124 bases and encodes several viral nonstructural proteins (e.g. methyltransferase, protease, helicase and RNA-dependent RNA polymerase). ORF2 contains 1980 bases at the 3′ end of the genome and encodes the viral capsid protein (CP).

ORF3, which partially overlaps with the other 2 ORFs, encodes a 13.5kDa regulatory phosphoprotein with multifunctions (Monga, 2011; Vasickova et al., 2007).
Due to the lack of a robust cell culture system, the viral structural studies have mainly relied on recombinant capsid protein (CP) from *in vitro* cell expression (Li et al., 2005; Li et al., 1997). Recent findings from HEV expression and purification, X-ray crystallography, and electron cryomicroscopy (cryoEM) have begun to shed new light on the structural and functional properties of this important human pathogen.

2. Hepatitis E virion morphology and capsid protein expression

Native hepatitis E viruses are a non-enveloped, spherically shaped particle. The viron is thought to be made of 180 copies of CP with an approximate diameter of 27-34nm (Guu et al., 2009; Xing et al., 1999). Both immune and negative stain electron microscopy of human stool specimens have showed that the diameter of HEV is about 32nm (Balayan et al., 1983; Bradley et al., 1988). The surface of the virion has obvious spikes that are slightly less pronounced than those of Norovirus, but is clearly distinct from the smooth, featureless surface of the hepatitis A virus (Guu et al., 2009; Xing et al., 2010). However, based on morphology alone, HEV could not be reliably distinguished from other small spherical human enteroviruses usually found in feces. The buoyant density of HEV particles was 1.35 to 1.40g/cm^3 in CsCl (Bradley et al., 1988).
Escherichia coli, and eukaryotic cell systems including insect, yeast and mammalian cells have been used to express the vrial capsid protein(CP). Among all of these *in vitro* cell systems, the baculovirus-insect cell system was proved to be an excellent choice to produce virus-like particles (VLPs) for its proper post-translational modification, correct conformation and assembly (Li et al., 2005; Li et al., 1997; Xing et al., 2011). In addition to the full-length 72-kDa protein predicted from the sequence of the ORF2 gene, abundant ORF2-related polypeptides with molecular weights of 53, 56, and 64 kDa were detected in the insect Sf9 and Tn5 cells (Fig1. A). The amino terminus of the 56.5- and 63-kDa proteins was amino acid 112, while the carboxy termini of these two proteins were found to be residue 607 and 635, respectively. There were also some conflicts on the exact site where the carboxy termini of these peptides end among different research groups. The molecular masses of HEV 53- and 56-kDa proteins were larger than expected from amino acid sequence possibly due to post-translational modifications
HEV CP could self-assemble into two populations of virus-like particles, a small one with a diameter of about 23 nm, and a large one with a diameter of about 42 nm (Fig. 1C and D). Although multiple polypeptides could be generated by expression of the full length ORF2 gene, only the 53-Kd peptide from aa 112 to aa 608 could self-assemble into the small particles. In contrast, the big particle was formed by the peptides from aa 14 to aa 608. The buoyant density of the small VLPs is only 1.285 g/cm^3 in CsCl gradient, and the large VLPs has a density of 1.31 g/cm^3 (Xing et al., 2010), both smaller than the buoyant densities of 1.35 g/cm^3 and 1.39 to 1.40 g/cm^3 reported for the native HEV particles extracted from in human stool possibly due to the lack of nucleic acids. In addition to the gene truncations at the N and C termini, the yield of HEV VLPs also depends on the insect cell lines used for overexpression. When using the Tn5 insect cells, the capsid proteins with 111 or 13 amino acids truncation at the N terminus could produce small or large particles at high yield (Li et al., 2005; Li et al., 1997; Xing et al., 2011).

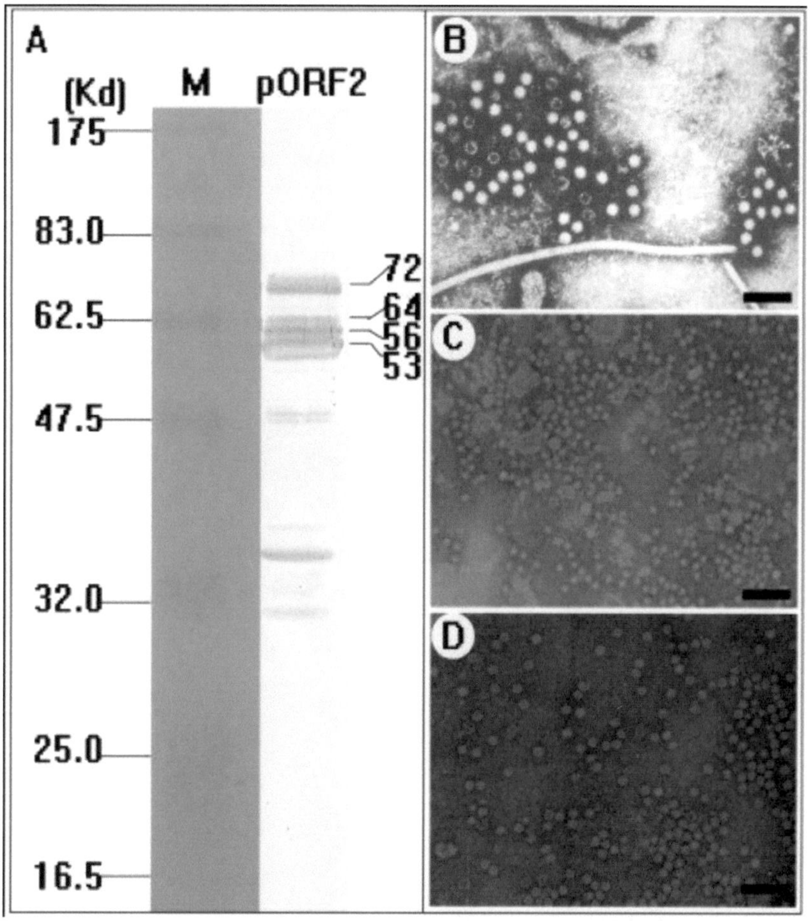

Fig. 1. Capsid protein and virions of HEV. (A) 10% SDS-PAGE of the full ORF2 proteins of genotype 4 from overexpression in Tn 5 cell. Target proteins were detected by western blot analysis using the serum of a patient with acute hepatitis E. M, molecular weight standard. (B) Native virions of hepatitis E virus under electron microscopy (Courtesy of Angusmclellan, CDC of United States). (C) Electron microscopy of small virus-like-particles (VLPs) (~23.7nm) purified from Tn5 cells by CsCl equilibrium centrifugation. The VLPs were stained with 2% phosphotungstic acid solution (buffered to pH 7 using sodium hydroxide). (D) Electron microscopy of large VLPs (~41.5nm) purified from Tn5 cells with CsCl equilibrium centrifugation. The VLPs were stained with 2% phosphotungstic acid solution (buffered to pH 7 using sodium hydroxide) Bar=100 Å.

3. The structure of small and large hepatitis E virus capsid

HEV VLPs made by the baculovirus-insect cell expression system are easy to purify to high concentration, thus making it possible for high resolution structural analyses. The structure of small VLPs has been analyzed first by cryoEM (Xing et al., 1999)and then by X-ray crystallography (Guu et al., 2009; Li et al., 2009; Yamashita et al., 2009). In the later case, the cryoEM map has served as a phasing model for crystal structure determination. In addition, the structure of large HEV VLPs has been extensively solved by electron cryomicroscopy (Xing et al., 2010). Our understanding of HEV capsid greatly benefited from the combination of medium-resolution cryoEM maps with atomic resolution X-ray crystal structures of these VLPs.

The cryoEM density map of the small VLP shows that the capsid consists of 60 copies of HEV CP arranged on T=1 lattice of icosahedral symmetry The capsid is decorated by a total of 30 dimeric protrusions each measured to be 56 Å long and 43 Å wide. These protrusions are found at twofold axes, with each protrusion surrounded by another four protrusions related by adjacent threefold axes (Fig2.B). Small plateaus are also found on threefold axes. Based on the cryoEM map, each CP molecule can be clearly divided into two domains, a shell domain and a protrusion domain (Fig2.B) (Li et al., 2005; Xing et al., 1999).

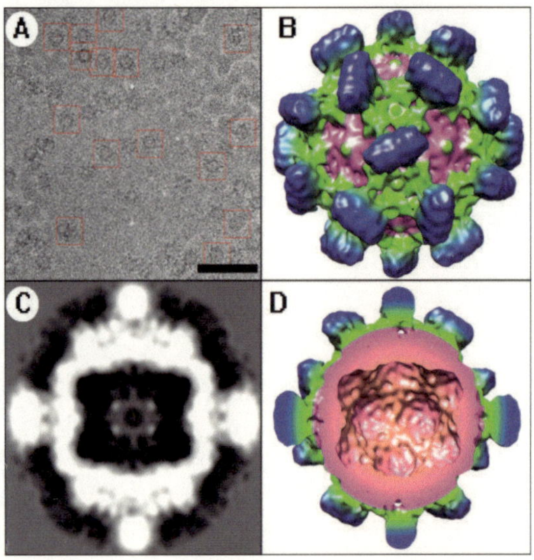

Fig. 2. The cryoEM structure of small VLPs. (A) CryoEM micrographs of small VLPs embedded in vitreous ice (Bar=1000 Å). (B) Shade surface of the small VLPs reconstruction at about 11-Å resolution as viewed along the twofold axis. The capsid is colored radially from inside to outside as magenta, green and blue, respectively. (C) A central slice view along the twofold axis. (D)Shade surface representation of the 3D reconstruction with tis upper half removed to reveal the internal feature.

Using the cryoEM reconstruction as phase model, the structure of the HEV small VLP was determined to atomic resolution by X-ray crystallography (Guu et al., 2009; Yamashita et al., 2009). In agreement with the low resolution density determined by cryoEM, the crystal structure of the *T=1* VLPs shows that each CP can be divided into 3 domains: the S domain (aa 118–313), the P1 domain (aa 314–453), and the P2 domain (aa 454–608) (Fig. 3A and B), with the latter two domains connected by a long, flexible hinge linker. The S domain forms a continuous capsid shell that is reinforced by 3-fold protrusions formed by P1 and 2-fold spikes formed by P2. The S domain adopts the jelly-roll, β-barrel fold that is most closely related to plant *T=3* viruses. Both P1 and P2 contain compact, 6-stranded barrels that resemble the β-barrel domain of phage sialidase and the receptor-binding domain of norovirus respectively (Guu et al.,2009). Although HEV CP contains 3 domains like the calicivirus coat protein, the organization of the 3 domains and their structural details are different (Fig. 3B). In calicivirus, the P2 domain is a large insertion in the P1 domain, while the 3 domains S, P1, and P2 are arranged in a linear sequence in *T=1* VLPs (Guu et al., 2009; Li et al., 2009; Yamashita et al., 2009).

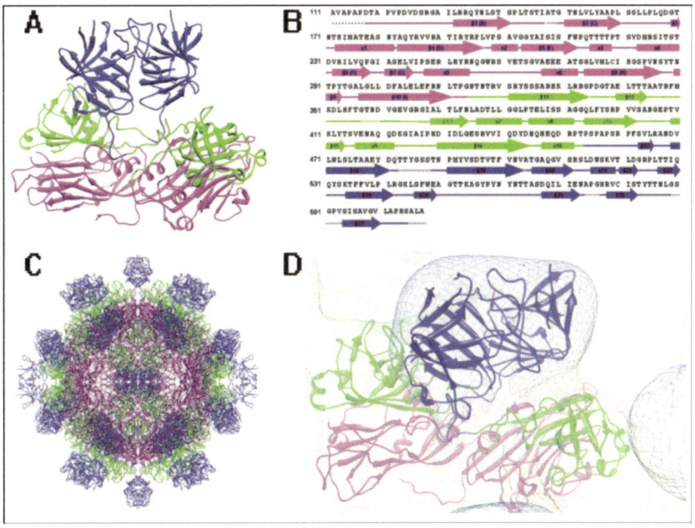

Fig. 3. The X-ray structure of small VLPs. (A) The ribbon diagram of a capsid monomer (PDB accession code: 2ZTN). The P2 (blue), P1 (green) and S (magenta) domains are at the top, middle, and bottom, respectively. (B) Secondary structure assignment. α-helices are shown by rectangles, β-strands by arrows, loops by thick lines, and disordered regions by dotted lines. Regions from the S, P1, and P2 domains are colored the same as in (A). The conventional naming scheme for the 8 β-strands (BIDG and CHEF) from the jelly-roll β-barrel is shown in parentheses. (C) The whole crystal structure of HEV *T=1* VLP. The three domains, S, P1, and P2 are similarly colored as in (A). (D) The crystal structure of one CP dimmer fits well into the cryoEM density of *T=3* VLP.

Meanwhile, the large VLPs have been proved that it is made up of 180 copied of coat protein. According to the cryoEM reconstruction of *T=3* VLPs (Xing et al., 2010), the density map reveals four discrete domains, P2, P1, S and N from outside to inward (Fig. 4C). The density profile of the P2, P1 and S domains displayed less variation from that observed in *T=1* VLPs, thus the CPs was able to be grouped into three unique monomers according to their geometric environments. Although monomers A and B formed dimeric spikes (A-B dimers) around each of the five-fold axes, two two-fold related C monomers formed a spike (C-C dimers) at each of the icosahedral two-fold axes (Fig. 4B). The surface lattices of CPs in *T=3* HEV-LP were similar to the capsid arrangement of caliciviruses. Comparing with the A-B dimer, the morphology of the HEV C-C dimer was less well defined, perhaps due to the flexibility in the angle of the protruding domain toward the icosahedral shell (Guu et al., 2009; Xing et al., 2010).

Although there is no crystal structure for the T=3 particles, a pseudo-atomic structure of the T=3 particles was obtained by docking the atomic structures of the CP from *T=1* particle into the T=3 cryoEM density map. The docking of the crystal structure of the T=1 CP to the density map of T=3 VLP showed very good agreement between the two structures (Fig. 3D). The docking positioned N-terminal tail of the HEV CP at the capsid inner surface and aligned well with an internal density linker in *T=3* VLPs. The linker density served as a tag to connect the N domain with the icosahedral capsid shell, highlighting the location of the N-terminal 111 amino acids of the HEV CP in the *T=3* VLP.

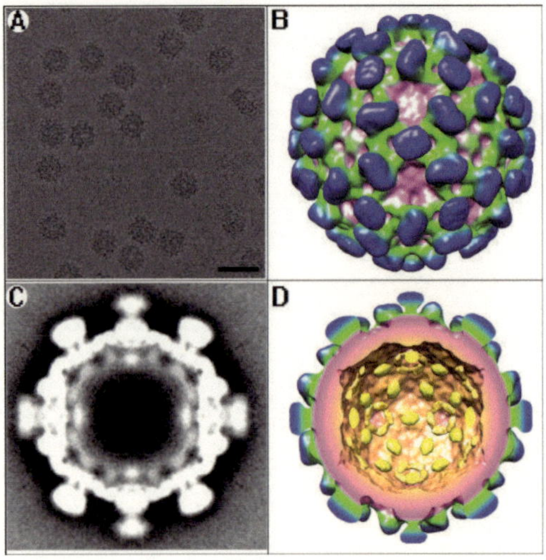

Fig. 4. CryoEM structure of the large VLPs. (A) CryoEM micrographs of large VLPs embedded in vitreous ice (Bar=1000 Å). (B) Shade surface of the large VLP reconstruction at about 11 Å resolution as viewed along the twofold axis (Electron Microscopy Data Bank accession number: EMD-5173). Different domains are colored differently, the S domain colored magenta, P1 domain green, P2 domain blue. (C) A central slice view along the twofold axis. (D) Shaded surface representation of the 3D reconstruction after its upper half was removed to reveal the internal view; the N domain is colored yellow.

4. Assembly mechanism of HEV capsids

After the structure of the *T=1* and *T=3* capsids of HEV were establised, it became possible to propose a model for the assembly of the capsids. Because HEV CP containing amino acids 112–608 self-assemble into T=1 VLP and CP containing amino acids 14–608 form T=3 VLP, it is likely that the N-arm acts as a molecular switch in regulating capsid assembly. Based on previous studies on the *T=3* viruses such as small plant RNA viruses, insect nodaviruses, and caliciviruses (Ban et al., 1995; Chen et al., 2006; Prasad et al., 1999), two different forms of dimers (A-B dimer and C-C dimer) are necessary for the formation of the *T=3* particles. Indeed, the *T=3* density map of HEV VLP confirms that it is composed of two types of dimmers: the angled A-B dimmer and the flat C-C dimmer. *In vitro*, dimer and decamer intermediates were found during the purification, disassembly and reassembly process. The finding of these CP assemblies helped us to understand the HEV capsid assembly process in some detail (Guu et al., 2009; Xing et al., 2010).

As for the *T=1* capsid, the CP monomers form stable dimers through the interactions largely mediated by P2 domain through an extended loop (550–566) and three β-strands from the central β-barrel. These CP dimers are designated A-B dimers and they are found on the icosahedral two-fold axis. The decamers, each assembled from five A-B dimers, are located at the 5-fold axes, and stabilized by interactions from four loops between the β-strands in

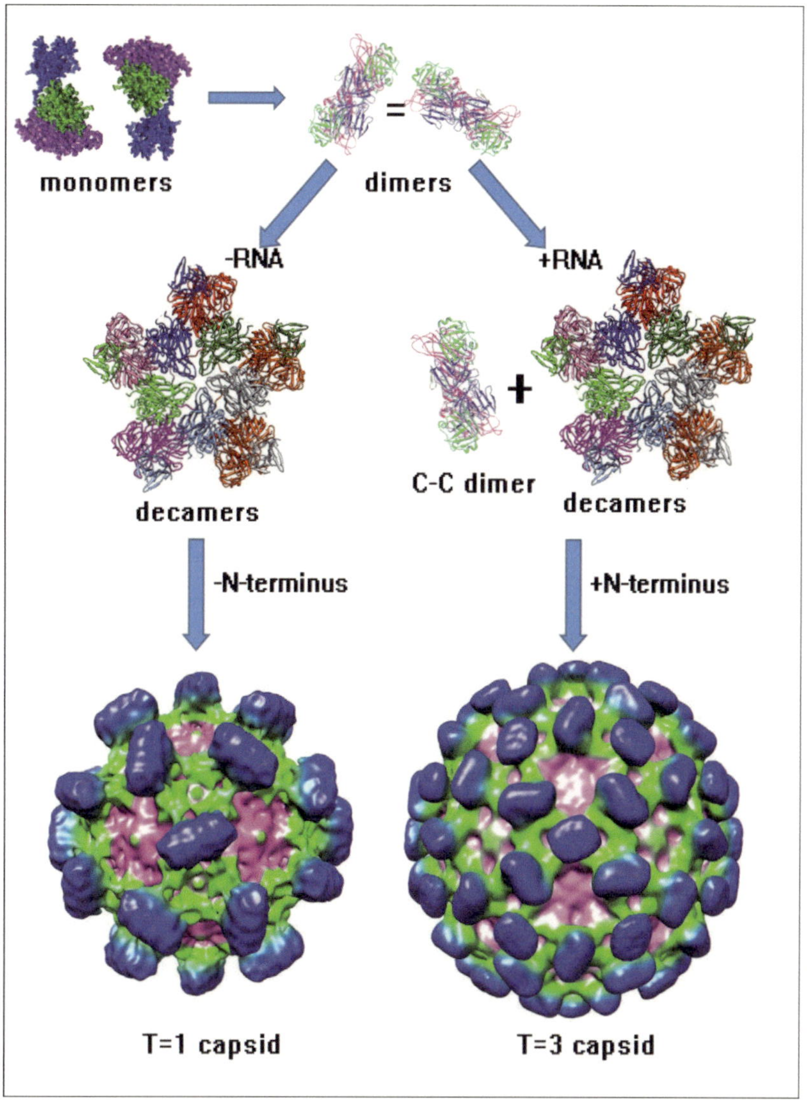

Fig. 5. Diagram showing the putative assembly process of HEV *T=1* and *T=3* VLPs. The HEV CP encodes information that controls the assembly of decamers. Interaction with the RNA fragment induces flat dimeric contact and the formation of C-C dimers, which guides the assembly of the complete T=3 icosahedral capsid.

the S domain. After formation of the decamers, they begin to interact around the three-fold axes to assemble the whole icosahedral capsid. Interactions around the three-fold protrusions are largely maintained by the P1 domains. In contrast to the formation of the *T=1* icosahedral capsid, *T=3* icosahedral capsid assembly utilizes a mechanism that requires the formation of the flat C-C dimmers help to assemble hexamers at icosahedral three-fold positions(Xing et al., 2010). The CP of *T=3* capsid has residues 14-118 at N terminus with an RNA binding activity. The induction of the C-C conformation was also noted in the bacteriophage MS2, where the complete assembly of capsid requires the presence of synthetic RNA fragment (Stockley et al., 2007). The interaction of RNA with the N-terminal end of ORF2 may act as the driving force leading the formation of flat C-C dimers and ultimately the full capsid formation through the integration of 30 copies of C-C dimmers and 12 copies of A-B decamers. One putative assembly model for *T=1* and *T=3* HEV capsids is depicted Figure 5.

5. Biological functions of HEV capsid and pathogenesis

Viral capsids help to provide structural support for the virion and to contain or protect the viral genome. In non-enveloped viruses, they also mediate cell receptor binding,virus internalization and viral genome release. In addition, viral capsids bind to antibodies and play important roles in inducing host immune reactions.

The three domains of VLP play different roles in organizing the icosahedral capsid. The S domain, which adopts the jelly-roll, β-barrel fold, forms a continuous capsid shell. The P1 domain interacts near three-fold axes, forming isolated trimetric protrusions. Thus, the P1 domain stabilizes only the trimetric interactions. The P2 domain forms dimeric spikes that stabilize capsid protein interactions across the two-folds (Guu et al., 2009; Li et al., 2009; Xing et al., 2010; Yamashita et al., 2009).

The two P domains play additional roles other than maintaining structural stability. The peptide of the HEV capsid protein (amino acids 368–606), which consists of a part of the P1 and entire P2 domain, was shown to be capable of binding and penetrating different cell lines susceptible to HEV, thus is capable of inhibiting HEV infection (He et al., 2008). The potential sugar binding sequence from the P1 domain, 376ADTLLGGLPTELISSA391, is strictly conserved among all HEV genotypes. In contrast, loops 550-566 and 583-593,the potential sugar binding site of the P2 domain, contain three and four hyper-variable amino acids, respectively, indicating that these regions are instead likely to mediate antibody recognition and immune escape. The putative sugar binding motif in the P1 domain (376–391) forms a hidden pocket at the interface between two capsid proteins around three-fold axes, suggesting receptor binding to P1 domain may potentially lead to the destabilization of the VLP trimer, resulting in conformational changes that eventually lead to membrane penetration and genome release into the infected cell. Further mutagenesis studies targeting these two potential sugar-binding sites will determine which domain functions in host-cell binding and virus internalization. Many studies also implicated the P1 and P2 domains in antibody binding (Guu et al., 2009; Li et al., 2009; Xing et al., 2010; Xing et al., 2011; Yamashita et al., 2009).

There are three potential N-glycosylation sites in the capsid protein that are well-conserved, Asn-137-Leu-Ser, Asn-310-Leu-Thr, and Asn-562-Thr-Thr. The N137 and N310 are hidden in the inside of the capsid. In the CP dimmer structure, these two sites are mapped on the horizontal surface of the S domain, suggesting that, if it occurs at all, N-glycosylation in these sites may inhibit assembly of VLPs. Indeed, Graff et al. reported that HEV carrying mutations in Asn-137 or Asn-310 to Glu lost infectivity to cells or rhesus macaques due to a defect in the virion assembly (Graff et al., 2008). N562 located at P2 domain is exposed to solvent at the very top of the surface spike, and could potentially be subjected to receive glycosylation in ER (Graff et al., 2008; Torresi et al., 1999).

The inner surface of the capsid shell is covered with a large number of basic amino acid side chains (R128, R133, R186, R189, R193, and R195, a total of six from each subunit), remarkably different from dsRNA viruses in which a large number of negatively charged residues on the inner surface are used to facilitate the movement of dsRNA genome during particle-associated transcription (Pan et al., 2009). These arginine side chains from capsids presumably help to neutralize the negative charges of the genomic RNA. Around the five-fold axes is a ring of five tyrosine residues (Y288) that are hydrogen bonded to five serine residues (S200), which are also positioned around the five-fold axes, but closer to the particle interior (Guu et al., 2009).

Presumably because the structural features of small HEV VLPs resemble that of the native virion, small VLPs possess antigenity similar to that of an authentic HEV particle and function as an antigen to detect HEV- specific immunoglobulin G (IgG) and immunoglobulin (IgM) responses (He et al., 2008; Xing et al., 1999; Xing et al., 2011; Yamashita et al., 2009). When VLPs are mixed and incubated with patient serum, the resultant antigen-antibody complexes are able to be examined under EM. Moreover, the VLPs can be also used as the antigen to detect HEV-specific antibodies elicited in an experimentally infected monkey, and obvious IgM and IgG antibody responses were observed during the clinical course of acute hepatitis. Oral administration of recombinant VLPs was immunogenic and stimulated an immune response in mice in the absence of an adjuvant, and all the antibody responses including IgM, IgG and IgA were obtained (Li et al., 2004; Li et al., 2001). Because of its large size and ability to encapsulate the viral genome,it is generally accepted that the T=3 VLPs have the same capside structure with native HEV. Therefore, the T=3 VLPs should have the same antigenic and immunological functions as the *T=1* VLPs as well as the native HEV virion.

6. Conclusion

Major advances have been achieved in the last few years in studying the structure and assembly of the hepatitis E virus capsid. Our structural and functional studies of HEV capsid have largely benefitted from the ability to produce large quantities of recombinant proteins, and under certain conditions to induce the assembly of the HEV-like particles. Many questions still remain unanswered, however. For example, what is the biological function of the C-terminal domain of the capsid protein? The C-terminal domain, or the last ~50 residues of the capsid protein, is not present in any of the virus-like particles that have been analyzed so far. It is possible that this sequence has an important role in HEV assembly but may not be needed for virus infectivity. The HEV cell receptor, which is recognized by the capsid protein, has not been identified either. Other interesting questions are how the infectious virion gets internalized into host cells, and subsequently how the capsid structure changes to release the viral genome into the host cytoplasm to initiate infection. It is anticipated that molecular virology together with structural biology methods such as cryo-EM and X-ray crystallography will continue to make important contributions to help answer these question. In the end, our ultimate understanding of the HEV capsid function requires an effective cell culture system where recombinant viruses can be generated and analyzed for virus entry, replication and growth.

7. Acknowledgments

We thank Drs. Ilker Donmez and Jinmin Cui for valuable discussions and Xiaokang Zhang and Jian He for preparing figure 5. Research in Drs. Zhang and Tao's laboratories was supported by Grants NO. 10274106 from Nation natrual funding of China (to JZ) and C-1565 from the Welch Foundation (to YJT).

8. References

Balayan, M. S.; Andjaparidze, A. G.; Savinskaya, S. S.; Ketiladze, E. S.; Braginsky, D. M.; Savinov, A. P. & Poleschuk, V. F. (1983). Evidence for a virus in non-A, non-B hepatitis transmitted via the fecal-oral route. Intervirology, 20, 1, pp.23-31, 0300-5526

Ban, N.; Larson, S. B. & McPherson, A. (1995). Structural comparison of the plant satellite viruses. Virology, 214, 2, pp.571-583, 0042-6822

Bradley, D.; Andjaparidze, A.; Cook, E. H.; McCaustland, K.; Balayan, M.; Stetler, H.; Velazquez, O.; Robertson, B.; Humphrey, C.; Kane, M. & Weisfuse, I. (1988). Aetiological agent of enterically transmitted non-A, non-B hepatitis. J Gen Virol, 69, pp.731-738, 0022-1317

Chen, R.; Neill, J. D.; Estes, M. K. & Prasad, B. V. V. (2006). X-ray structure of a native calicivirus: Structural insights into antigenic diversity and host specificity. Proc Natl Acad Sci U S A, 103, 21, pp.8048-8053, 0027-8424

Fauquet, C. M.; Mayo, M. A.; Maniloff, J.; Desselberger, U. & Ball, L. A. Eds. (2005). Virus taxonomy: VIIIth report of the International Committee on Taxonomy of Viruses, Elsevier Academic Press, 0122499514, San Diego

Graff, J.; Zhou, Y. H.; Torian, U.; Nguyen, H.; Claire, M. S.; Yu, C.; Purcell, R. H. & Emerson, S. U. (2008). Mutations within potential glycosylation sites in the capsid protein of hepatitis E virus prevent the formation of infectious virus particles. J. Virol., 82, 3, pp.1185-1194, 0022-538X

Guu, T. S. Y.; Liu, Z.; Ye, Q. Z.; Mata, D. A.; Li, K. P.; Yin, C. C.; Zhang, J. Q. & Tao, Y. J. (2009). Structure of the hepatitis E virus-like particle suggests mechanisms for virus assembly and receptor binding. Proc Natl Acad Sci U S A, 106, 31, pp.12992-12997, 0027-8424

He, S. Z.; Miao, J.; Zheng, Z. Z.; Wu, T.; Xie, M. H.; Tang, M.; Zhang, J.; Ng, M. H. & Xia, N. S. (2008). Putative receptor-binding sites of hepatitis E virus. J Gen Virol, 89, pp.245-249, 0022-1317

Hochman, J. A. & Balistreri, W. F. (1999). Viral hepatitis: expanding the alphabet. Adv Pediatr, 46, pp.207-43, 0065-3101

Knipe, D. M.; Howley, P. M.; Griffin, D. E.; Lamb, R. A.; Martin, M. A.; Roizman, B. & Straus, S. E. Eds. (2007). Fields Virology, Lippincott Williams & Wilkins, 0781760607, Philadelphia

Kumar, V.; Das, S. & Jameel, S. (2010). The biology and pathogenesis of hepatitis viruses. Curr Sci, 98, 3, pp.312-325, 0011-3891

Li, S.; Tang, X.; Seetharaman, J.; Yang, C.; Gu, Y.; Zhang, J.; Du, H.; Shih, J.; Hew, C.; Sivaraman, J. & Xia, N. (2009). Dimerization of Hepatitis E virus capsid protein E2s domain is essential for virus-host interaction. PLoS Pathog, 5:e1000537

Li, T. C.; Suzaki, Y.; Ami, Y.; Dhole, T. N.; Miyamura, T. & Takeda, N. (2004). Protection of cynomolgus monkeys against HEV infection by oral administration of recombinant hepatitis E virus-like particles. Vaccine, 22, 3-4, pp.370-377, 0264-410X

Li, T. C.; Takeda, N. & Miyamura, T. (2001). Oral administration of hepatitis E virus-like particles induces a systemic and mucosal immune response in mice. Vaccine, 19, 25-26, pp.3476-3484, 0264-410X

Li, T. C.; Takeda, N.; Miyamura, T.; Matsuura, Y.; Wang, J. C. Y.; Engvall, H.; Hammar, L.; Xing, L. & Cheng, R. H. (2005). Essential elements of the capsid protein for self-assembly into empty virus-like particles of hepatitis E virus. J. Virol., 79, 20, pp.12999-13006, 0022-538X

Li, T. C.; Yamakawa, Y.; Suzuki, K.; Tatsumi, M.; Razak, M. A. A.; Uchida, T.; Takeda, N. & Miyamura, T. (1997). Expression and self-assembly of empty virus-like particles of hepatitis E virus. J. Virol., 71, 10, pp.7207-7213, 0022-538X

Meng, X. J. (2010). Recent advances in Hepatitis E Virus. J Viral Hepat, 17, 3, pp.153-161, 1352-0504

Monga, S. P. S. Ed. (2011). Molecular Pathology of Liver Diseases, Springer, 9781441971067, New York

Okamoto, H. (2007). Genetic variability and evolution of hepatitis E virus. Virus Res., 127, 2, pp.216-228, 0168-1702

Pan, J. H.; Dong, L. P.; Lin, L.; Ochoa, W. F.; Sinkovits, R. S.; Havens, W. M.; Nibert, M. L.; Baker, T. S.; Ghabrial, S. A. & Tao, Y. Z. J. (2009). Atomic structure reveals the unique capsid organization of a dsRNA virus. Proc Natl Acad Sci U S A, 106, 11, pp.4225-4230, 0027-8424

Panda, S. K.; Thakral, D. & Rehman, S. (2007). Hepatitis E virus. Rev Med Virol. , 17, 3, pp.151-180, 1052-9276

Prasad, B. V. V.; Hardy, M. E.; Dokland, T.; Bella, J.; Rossmann, M. G. & Estes, M. K. (1999). X-ray crystallographic structure of the Norwalk virus capsid. Science, 286, 5438, pp.287-290, 0036-8075

Reyes, G. R., Purdy, M. A., Kim, J. P., Luk, K. C., Young, L. M., Fry, K. E. &Bradley, D. W. (1990). Isolation of a cDNA from the virus responsible for enterically transmitted non-A, non-B hepatitis. Science 247, pp1335–1339

Stockley, P. G.; Rolfsson, O.; Thompson, G. S.; Basnak, G.; Francese, S.; Stonehouse, N. J.; Homans, S. W. & Ashcroft, A. E. (2007). A simple, RNA-mediated allosteric switch controls the pathway to formation of a T=3 viral capsid. J Mol Biol, 369, 2, pp.541-552, 0022-2836

Takahashi, M.; Tanaka, T.; Takahashi, H.; Hoshino, Y.; Nagashima, S.; Jirintai; Mizuo, H.; Yazaki, Y.; Takagi, T.; Azuma, M.; Kusano, E.; Isoda, N.; Sugano, K. & Okamoto, H. (2010). Hepatitis E Virus (HEV) Strains in Serum Samples Can Replicate Efficiently in Cultured Cells Despite the Coexistence of HEV Antibodies: Characterization of HEV Virions in Blood Circulation. J Clin Microbiol, 48, 4, pp.1112-1125, 0095-1137

Tam, A. W.; Smith, M. M.; Guerra, M. E.; Huang, C. C.; Bradley, D. W.; Fry, K. E. & Reyes, G. R. (1991). Hepatitis E virus (HEV): molecular cloning and sequencing of the full-length viral genome. Virology, 185, 1, pp.120-131, 0042-6822

Torresi, J.; Li, F.; Locarnini, S. A. & Anderson, D. A. (1999). Only the non-glycosylated fraction of hepatitis E virus capsid (open reading frame 2) protein is stable in mammalian cells. J Gen Virol, 80, pp.1185-1188, 0022-1317

Vasickova, P.; Psikal, I.; Kralik, P.; Widen, F.; Hubalek, Z. & Pavlik, I. (2007). Hepatitis E virus: a review. Vet. Med.-Czech, 52, 9, pp.365-384, 0375-8427

Xing, L.; Kato, K.; Li, T. C.; Takeda, N.; Miyamura, T.; Hammar, L. & Cheng, R. H. (1999). Recombinant hepatitis e capsid protein self-assembles into a dual-domain T=1 particle presenting native virus epitopes. Virology, 265, 1, pp.35-45, 0042-6822

Xing, L.; Li, T. C.; Mayazaki, N.; Simon, M. N.; Wall, J. S.; Moore, M.; Wang, C. Y.; Takeda, N.; Wakita, T.; Miyamura, T. & Cheng, R. H. (2010). Structure of Hepatitis E Virion-sized Particle Reveals an RNA-dependent Viral Assembly Pathway. J Biol Chem, 285, 43, pp.33175-33183, 0021-9258

Xing, L.; Wang, J. C.; Li, T.-C.; Yasutomi, Y.; Lara, J.; Khudyakov, Y.; Schofield, D.; Emerson, S. U.; Purcell, R. H.; Takeda, N.; Miyamura, T. & Cheng, R. H. (2011). Spatial Configuration of Hepatitis E Virus Antigenic Domain. J Virol, 85, 2, 0022-538X(print) | 1098-5514(electronic)

Yamashita, T.; Mori, Y.; Miyazaki, N.; Cheng, R. H.; Yoshimura, M.; Unno, H.; Shima, R.; Moriishi, K.; Tsukihara, T.; Li, T. C.; Takeda, N.; Miyamura, T. & Matsuura, Y. (2009). Biological and immunological characteristics of hepatitis E virus-like particles based on the crystal structure. Proc Natl Acad Sci U S A, 106, 31, pp.12986-12991, 0027-8424